Peripheral Vascular Doppler Ultrasound Testing with Nutrition and Exercise for PAD

John A. Allocca, D.Sc., Ph.D.

Published by
Allocca Biotechnology, LLC
New York
www.allocca.com

Printed by createspace.com

ISBN 978-1-499-64042-7

Table of Contents

Introduction

Reducing the risk factors that lead to peripheral artery disease is critical to stop progression, such as reducing cholesterol and blood pressure, not smoking, and eating a healthy low fat diet. Aspirin may be prescribed or other anti-clotting drugs. The most effective treatment is exercise. In cases of severe peripheral artery disease, surgery can bypass a blocked artery and restore blood flow. Peripheral artery disease is dangerous, even when it's silent. Even when symptoms are not noticeable, people with peripheral artery disease decrease their activity level over time. Peripheral artery disease is proof that atherosclerosis is occurring throughout the body. Even if peripheral artery disease never causes problems itself, it increases the risk of dying from heart attack or stroke significantly.

Doppler ultrasound devices are used to measure the blood flowing in peripheral arteries. Peripheral artery disease (PAD) occurs when the blood vessels become narrow from the build up of plaque along the artery walls, which is referred to as atherosclerosis. PAD most commonly occurs in the legs, feet, and toes.

One in 12 U.S. service members who died in the Iraq and Afghanistan wars had plaque buildup in the arteries around their hearts - an early sign of heart disease, according to a new study. "Earlier autopsy studies... were critical pieces of information that alerted the medical community to the lurking burden of coronary disease in our young people," said Dr. Daniel Levy, director of the Framingham Heart Study and a senior investigator with the National Institutes of Health. Altogether the researchers had information on 3,832 service members who'd been killed at an average age of 26. Close to 9 percent had any buildup in their coronary arteries, according to the autopsies. And about a quarter of the soldiers with buildup in their arteries had severe blockage.

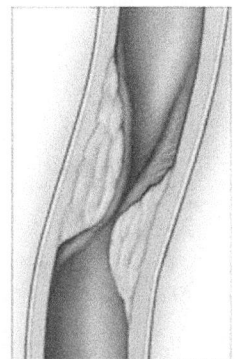

Artery narrowed by plaque

Hemodynamics

The circulatory system consists of a system of a pump (the heart), arteries, microcirculation, and venous return. The heart generates a pulsating flow of blood. Blood leaves the heart from the left ventricle through the aorta. Then, through smaller arteries. Then, through arterioles and capillaries where oxygen, glucose, etc. is transferred to the cells. The capillaries connect to the venues were carbon dioxide is picked up. The blood travels through a network of veins and into the heart through the inferior vena cava (from the body) and superior vena cava (from the head) to the right atrium. From the right atrium it is pumped into the right ventricle. Then, the blood is pumped to the lungs through the pulmonary artery to exchange carbon dioxide and oxygen. Then, back to the heart through the pulmonary vein into the left atrium. From the left atrium, blood is pumped into the left ventricle. Then, out into the aorta. Note the pulmonary artery is the only artery in the body that contains deoxygenated blood and the pulmonary vein is the only vein in the body that contains oxygenated blood. Resistance occurs primarily from the arterioles and somewhat from the capillaries.

Factors influencing hemodynamics are carbon dioxide, circulating blood volume, respiration, vascular diameter, resistance, and blood viscosity. It may also be influenced by diet, exercise, disease, drugs or alcohol, obesity and excess weight.

The loss of resistance of blood flow occurs from friction between the blood and blood vessel wall.

Changes in blood pressure and blood flow occurs from the acceleration of blood flow with systole and deceleration in diastole as the heart pumps in a pulsate pattern.

Arterial obstruction or narrowing (stenosis) results in reduced pressure and blood flow distal from the obstruction. However, the effects of obstruction also effect the blood pressure and blood flow proximal to the obstruction. Arteries offer very little resistance to flow. Obstructions must be substantial in order to affect blood flow distal from the obstruction. The effect of stenosis is seen more in the peripheral arteries.

Low pressure may be seen in mild stenosis when the patient is at rest. The presence of mild stenosis can be seen if blood flow is increased with exercise. The increase of blood flow though the stenosis results in a loss of energy due to friction distal to the stenosis.

The presence of severe stenosis may not be seen at rest because of the development of collateral circulation and a possible decrease in peripheral resistance.

Blood blow during exercise can increase in the muscles of the extremity distal to a stenosis. However, the distal pressure is reduced during exercise, muscles may draw blood from the skin of the foot resulting in numbness of the foot. This is a common symptom of claudication.

The pressure in the veins after blood flow in the arteriole and capillaries is about that of atmospheric pressure for a patient at rest in the supine position. Veins have relative large diameters and offer little resistance to blood flow. The effects of arterial pressure and blood flow are rarely transmitter to the systemic veins. However, phasic changes venous pressure and blood flow reflect changes in the right atrium pressures in response to cardiac activity.

Posture has an effect on pressure in veins. In the upright position, the pressure is increased in the lower extremities and leads to vascular distention.

The movement of the muscles in the legs leads to a decrease in venous pressure because of the one way values in the peripheral veins. The contraction of muscles squeeze the veins and cause the blood to flow towards the heart.

Venous thrombosis may lead to to a potentially fatal pulmonary embolism due to embolization of thrombi in the leg veins and resulting obstruction of the pulmonary arteries. Venous ultrasound is the primary means of diagnosis. Severe obstruction can lead to edema. A Doppler sound over the peripheral vein is present. Venous sounds are distinguished from arterial sounds by the absence of pulsate flow and the respiratory wind storm sound. Squeezing the limb distal to the site should temporally increase blood flow and cause an audible augmentation sound in the vein.

Various doppler plethysmographic methods can detect the rate of venous filling by measuring the changes in venous volume after the blood volumes have been decreased during muscular action of flexion extension of the ankle in the upright position.

Doppler Physics

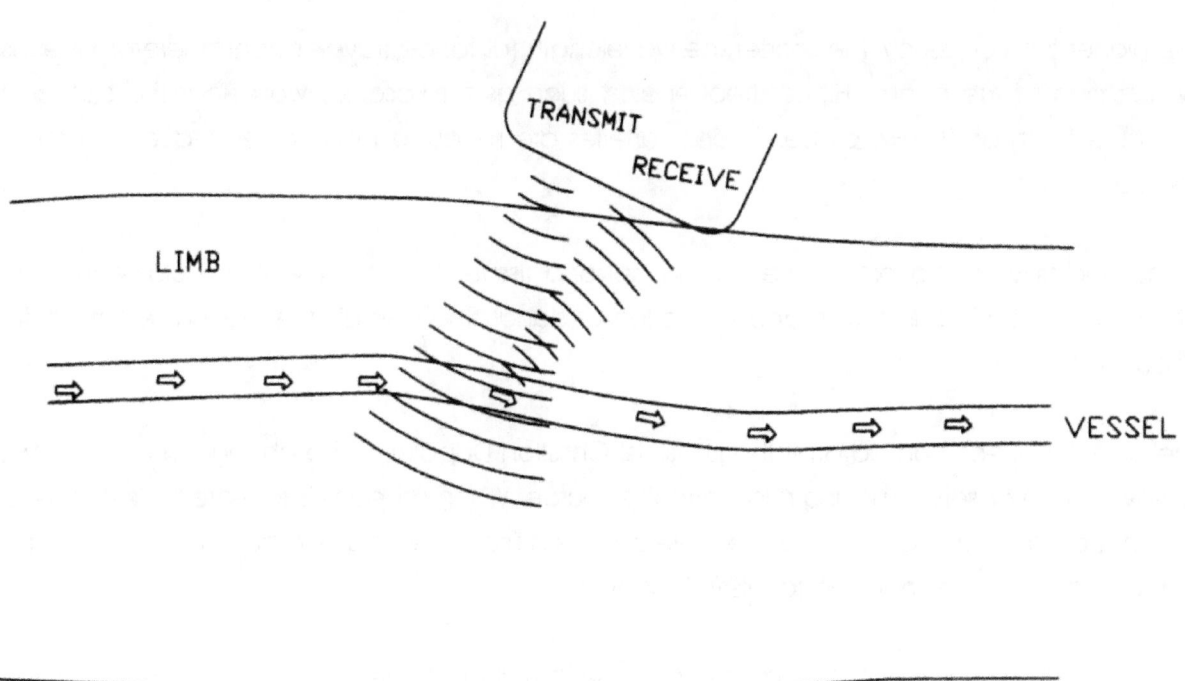

Frequency is expressed as Hertz, named after the physicist Heinrich Rudolf Hertz. It was formerly expressed as cycles per second. The wavelength is the length of one complete cycle. Velocity is expressed in cm/sec.

Velocity = frequency (Hertz symbolized as Hz) x wavelength (meters symbolized as m).

The longer the wavelength, the lower the frequency and vica versa .

The range of human hearing is 20 to 20,000 (20 KHz).

The range of ultrasound is 2.5 to 14,000,000 (14 MHz).

The velocity of sound in air is 330 meter/sec (m/s)

The velocity of sound in water is 1,500 meter/sec (m/s).

Gel is used to conduct ultrasound waves because the velocity is faster in water than air. Piezoelectricity is the effect of generating electricity from pressure applied to a crystal. In the doppler probe, a crystalline material is inserted into the head. When electric current is applied, the crystalline material vibrates at a frequency that is specific for that crystal. The vibrations are transmitted through tissue as ultrasound waves. The sound waves bounce back from the tissue towards the probe. The sound waves cause the crystal in the probe to vibrate and generate an electric current.

The higher the frequency, the shorter the wavelength (distance traveled) and therefore the less penetration of the beam. Higher frequencies, such as for vascular work near the surface is measured with an 8 MHz. probe. Deeper arteries are measured with lower frequency probes, such as 4 MHz.

Ultrasound travels at a precise velocity in gel and tissue. The instrument calculates the time elapsed between transmission and reception of signal. The crystals precisely differentiate the direction of the reflected signals.

The doppler effect, named after the physicist Christian Doppler, is the change in frequency of a wave for an observer moving relative to the source. When a beam is reflected, it's frequency will change as a function of distance traveled. This is like the sound of a train that gets lower as it approaches and higher as it travels further away.

This is the same principle that radar uses at a much higher frequency.

Doppler Sounds

The first long sound is from the systolic forward flow velocity.

The second short sound is from the reverse flow the baseline (closure of Aortic valve).

The third short sound is from arterial wall motion and is characteristic of a compliant artery.

Arteries of the Extremities

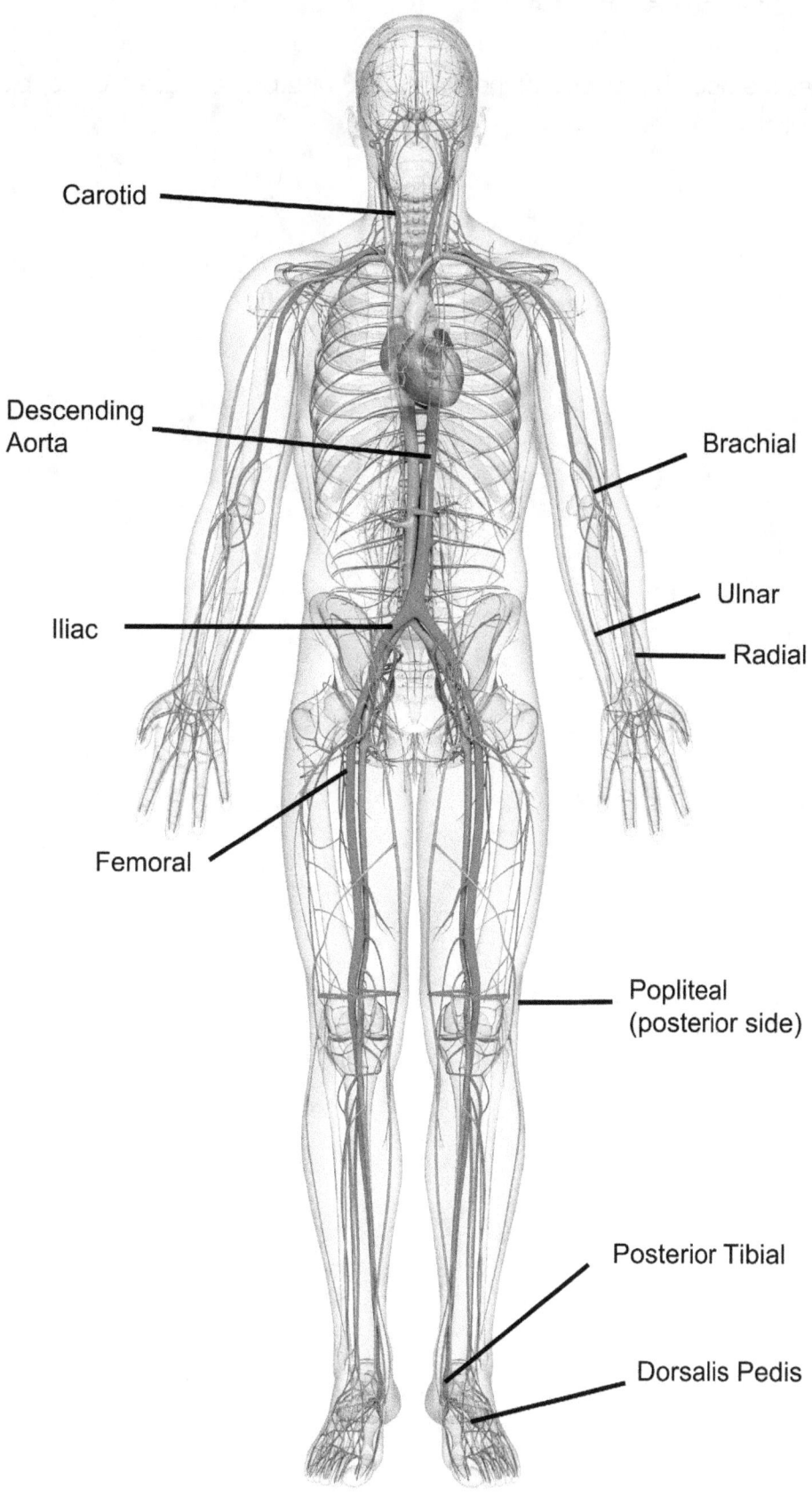

Carotid

Descending Aorta

Iliac

Femoral

Brachial

Ulnar

Radial

Popliteal
(posterior side)

Posterior Tibial

Dorsalis Pedis

The arteries that are used with doppler measurement are either the Brachial artery in the arm or true radical artery in the wrist, the Posterior Tibial artery at the medial side of the ankle, and the Dorsalis Pedis artery on the top of the foot.

These arteries are near the surface of the limbs. An 8 MHz probe is used for doppler ultrasound at these locations.

Waveform Analysis

The ultrasonic or doppler waveform follows the blood flow pulse of arteries. The analyses ultrasonic or doppler waveforms provide information for assessing the extent and location of peripheral vascular disease. The normal waveform is triphasic and includes forward and reverse (diastolic) components. With progression of disease, the reverse component is lost, and the waveform becomes biphasic. When forward flow becomes continuous, the waveform is considered monophasic. In severe disease, the waveform amplitude is dampened.

Characteristics of a doppler arterial waveform

1. A sharp rise in the upstroke representing the systolic pulse.
2. A more gradual decline during diastole, sometimes with bowing during diastole.
3. A dicrotic notch in the diastolic down stroke in waveforms of blood vessels close to the heart, such as the carotid and brachial arteries will show the dichotic notch (the closing of the aortic valve) in a healthy individual.

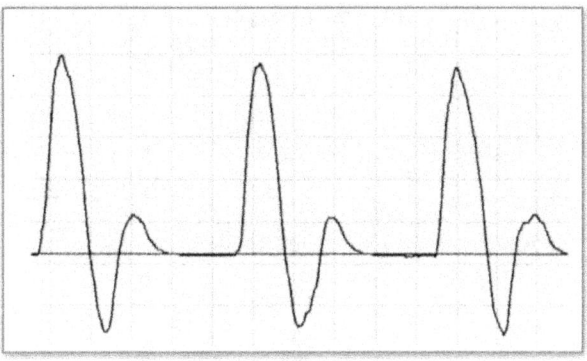

Normal Resting (Triphasic)

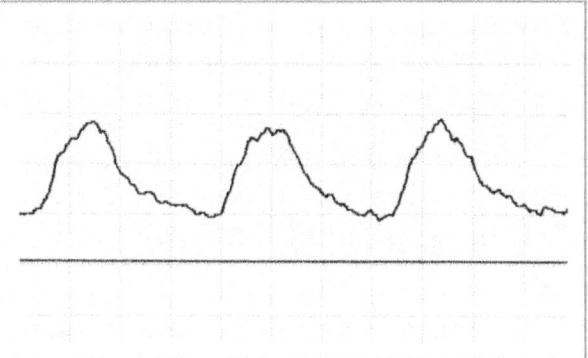

Early diastolic flow reversal (Biphasic)

Prolonged systolic upstroke, pandiastolic forward flow without diastolic flow reversal (monophasic)

Ankle Brachial Index (ABI)

The ankle-brachial index (ABI) is a standard that is used to diagnose and predict the severity of peripheral arterial disease.

Calculate Ankle Brachial Index (ABI)

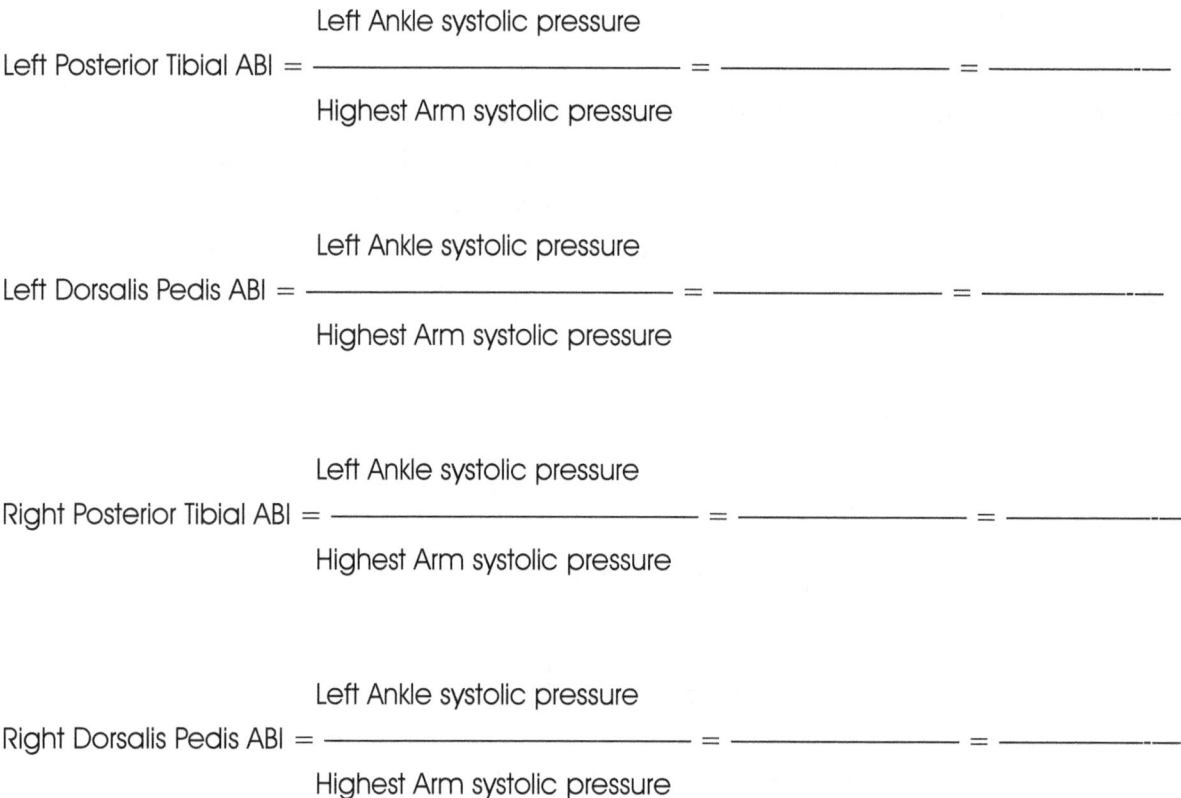

Left Posterior Tibial ABI = $\dfrac{\text{Left Ankle systolic pressure}}{\text{Highest Arm systolic pressure}}$ = —————— = ——————

Left Dorsalis Pedis ABI = $\dfrac{\text{Left Ankle systolic pressure}}{\text{Highest Arm systolic pressure}}$ = —————— = ——————

Right Posterior Tibial ABI = $\dfrac{\text{Left Ankle systolic pressure}}{\text{Highest Arm systolic pressure}}$ = —————— = ——————

Right Dorsalis Pedis ABI = $\dfrac{\text{Left Ankle systolic pressure}}{\text{Highest Arm systolic pressure}}$ = —————— = ——————

ABI / Severity of Disease:
> 1.40 = Noncompressible
1.00 - 1.40 = Normal
0.91 - 0.99 = Borderline
0.00 - 0.90 = Abnormal
Creager MA, et al. (2011). 2012 ACCF/AHA/ACR/SCAI/SIR/STS/SVM/SVN

Brachial Artery Pressure for Ankle Brachial Index (ABI) Study

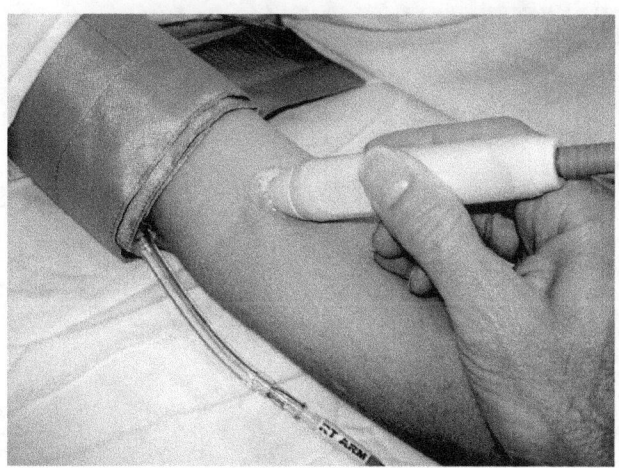

1. Have the patient rest horizontally for 5 minutes.

2. Place 12 cm blood pressure cuffs on the arms and the 10 cm cuffs on the ankles. Do not inflate the cuffs at this time.

3. Place ultrasound gel on the skin above the left brachial artery as shown above.

4. Gently place the Doppler probe over the left brachial artery. Do not apply pressure. Hold the probe above the artery at a 45 to 60 degree angle against flow. Adjust the probe angle until the best sound is heard and a steady waveform appears on the LCD.

5. Record the type of waveform on the ABI Form (Triphasic, Biphasic, Monophasic).

6. Take the systolic pressure by inflating the cuff to 20 mmHg over pressure (sound) cessation. Then, slowly deflate the cuff at a rate of 2-3 mmHg per second until the first Doppler sound is heard and waveform motion on the LCD returns.

7. Record the pressure on the ABI Form.

8. Repeat steps 3 through 8 for the right brachial artery.

Note: It doesn't matter if you start on the left of the right.

Posterior Tibial Artery Waveform and Pressure for ABI Study

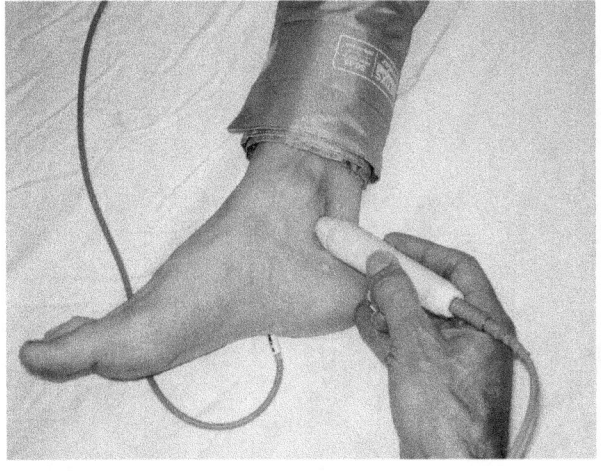

Posterior Tibial Artery

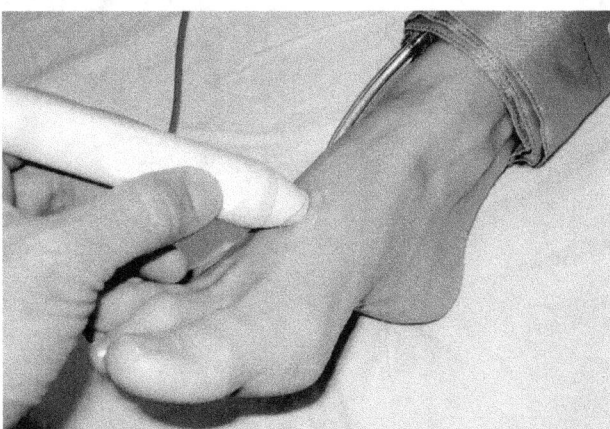

Dorsalis Pedis Artery

1. Apply ultrasound gel to the skin above the left posterior tibial artery as shown above.

2. Gently place the Doppler probe over the left posterior tibial artery. Do not apply pressure. Hold the probe above the artery at a 45 to 60 degree angle against flow. Adjust the probe angle until the best sound is heard and a steady waveform appears on the LCD. If waveform cannot be obtained from the left Posterior Tibial, use the left Dorsalis Pedis artery.

3. Record the type of waveform on the ABI Form (Triphasic, Biphasic, Monophasic).

4. Print the waveform.

5. Take the systolic pressure by inflating the cuff to 20 mmHg over pressure (sound) cessation. Then, slowly deflate the cuff at a rate of 2-3 mmHg per second until the first Doppler sound is heard and waveform motion on the LCD returns.

6. Record the pressure on the ABI Form.

7. Repeat steps 1 trough 6 for the right posterior tibial artery.

Note: It doesn't matter if you start on the left of the right.

Segmental Pressures Study

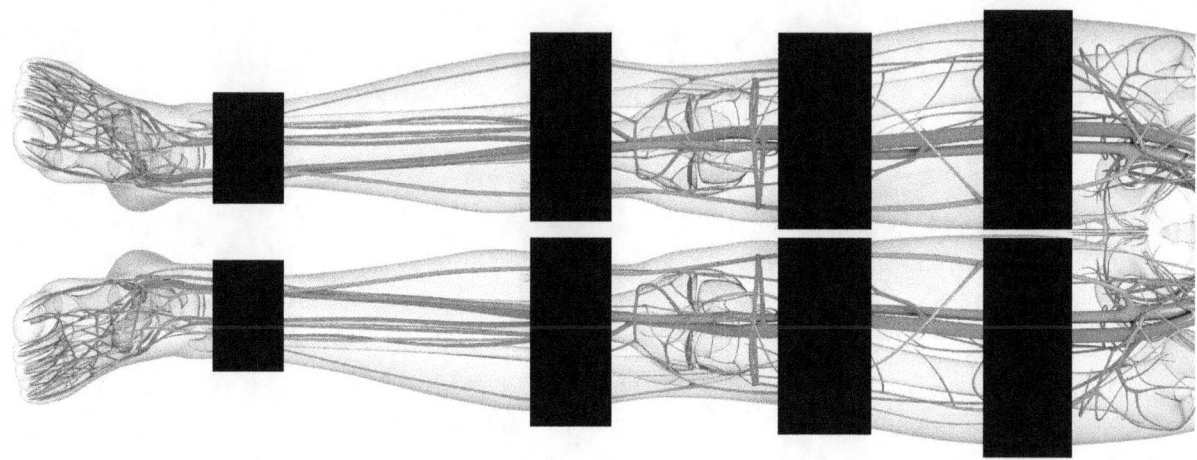

Segmental pressure study is used to measure the systolic pressure at different levels in the legs to evaluate blood flow and identify the location of blockages in the leg. Significant pressure differences between cuffs indicates a narrowing of an artery or blockage.

1. Place the patient in a supine position.

2. Place cuffs at high thigh, above and below the knee and the ankle.

3. Before taking systolic pressures at the leg, print the waveforms at the Posterior Tibial, Dorsalis pedis, popliteal, and femoral arteries.

4. Apply ultrasound gel to the skin above the left posterior tibial artery as shown above.

5. Gently place the Doppler probe over each arterial segment to be measured. Hold the probe above the artery at a 45 to 60 degree angle against flow. Adjust the probe angle until the best sound is heard and a steady waveform appears on the LCD.

6. Take the systolic pressure by inflating the cuff to 20 mmHg over pressure (sound) cessation. Then, slowly deflate the cuff at a rate of 2-3 mmHg per second until the first Doppler sound is heard and waveform motion on the LCD returns.

7. Record the pressure at posterior tibial, dorsalis pedis, popliteal, and femoral arteries.

8. Repeat on the other leg.

8. Significant pressure differences of 20 mm Hg or greater between cuffs indicates a narrowing of the artery or blockage.

Toe Brachial Index (TBI) Toe Pressure Study

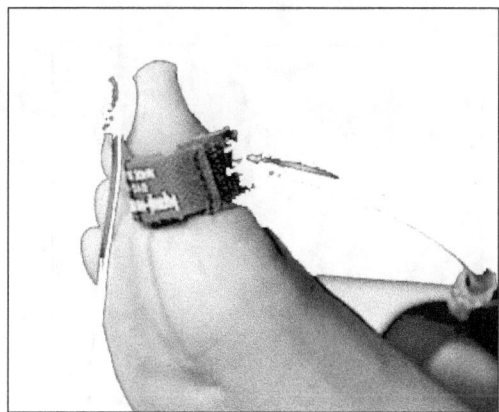

Toe brachial index study is used in unsuspected vascular disease and diabetes. In this study, infrared is used instead of ultrasound. Toe pressures are useful in cases of unsuspected vascular disease and in baseline diabetic type 2 foot where falsely high ankle pressures can occur due to calcification. Toe pressures are also useful in studying ulcer-healing potential in the diabetic foot.

1. Place the patient in a supine position so that the toe is at the same level as the heart.

2. Be sure that the room temperature is comfortable and that the skin surface of the toe is warm because cold constricts the superficial blood vessels and may affect the accuracy of the PPG measurements.

3. Place the digit cuff around the base of the toe

4. Place the PPG sensor to the pad of the toe using double sided clear tape or a velcro strap.

5. Take the systolic pressure by inflating the cuff to 20 mmHg over pressure (sound) cessation. Then, slowly deflate the cuff at a rate of 2-3 mmHg per second until the first Doppler sound is heard and waveform motion on the LCD returns.

6. Record the pressure.

7. Calculate TBI:
   TBI = Toe Pressure / Highest Arm Pressure.
   TBI > 0.7 = Normal.
   TBI <= 0.7 = Abnormal

8. Repeat on the other leg.

Venous Reflux Study

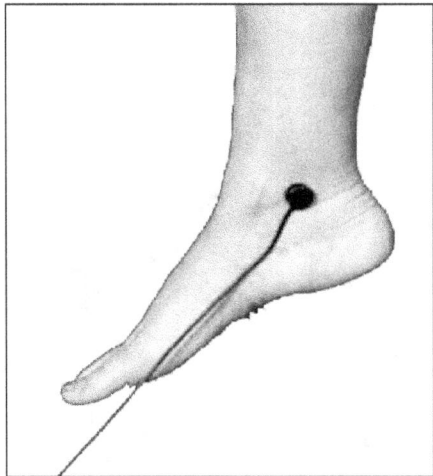

The venous reflux study is used to access for valvular competence. Recording time (RT) is venous refill time. Proper technique and patient cooperation are important factors in this study.

1. Before beginning the test, instruct the patient how to dorsiflex the foot using the calf muscle as a pump.

2. Set the doppler for DC Mode and Count 5x.

3. Place the PPG probe above the posterior tibial artery at or above the ankle.

4. Switch module to PPG setting.

5. Place the patient in a sitting position.

6. Press the probe button or right arrow button to activate the timer.

7. Ask the patient to dorsiflex the foot the number of times following the foot on the LCD screen.

8. Rest the foot.

9. Observe waveform on the LCD display, which will show a steady motion upward towards the baseline. When the test is complete the doppler will freeze and print the results including the recovery time.

10. The test may be repeated by placing a vascular cuff above knee and inflating it to 60 mmHg to rule out superficial venous reflux and direct augmentation of deep veins.

11. The patient should be referred for duplex imaging if the recovery time is marginal, less than

18 seconds or displays other symptoms according to the judgement of the physician.

RT > 21 = normal.

RT 18-21 = questionable - repeat test.

< 18 = venous reflux disease.

Pulse Volume Arterial Studies (PVR)

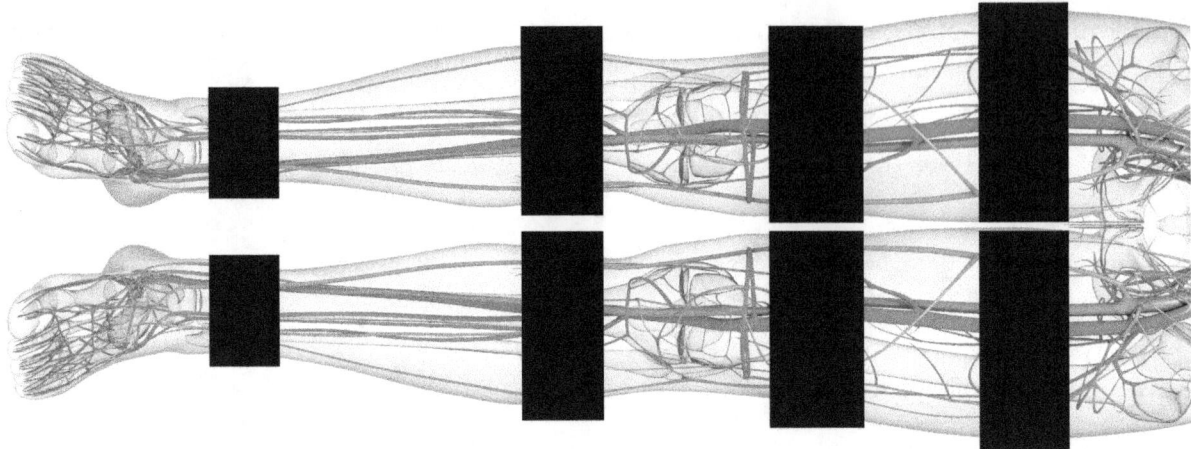

Pulse volume arterial study uses pneumoplethysmography or pulse volume to identify changes in leg blood volume through waveform pattern analysis and pulse contour criteria. PVRs are used in patients where vessel calcification presents inaccurate Doppler signal processing and falsely elevated pressure measurements.

1. Place the patient into the supine position.

2. Cuffs at high thigh, above and below the knee and the ankle.

3. On the PVC module switch to PV.

4. Set the doppler for AC Mode.

5. Connect a 3-way stopcock to the inlet of the PV module. Connect extender tubing to one of the two remaining sides of the stopcock and attach the tubing to one of the cuffs. Attach a sphygmomanometer to the other side of the stopcock.

6. Turn the stopcock so that air is routed from the sphygmomanometer to the cuff. The green arms on the stopcock will be at the 12, 3, and 6 o'clock positions.

7. Inflate cuff to 60 mHg.

8. Print the waveform.

9. Deflate the cuff and repeat for other cuffs.

10. The general method of interpreting PV waveforms by pattern recognition. A normal PV arterial waveform will display a rapid rise in the upstroke during systole and a sharp peak at maximum amplitude, followed by a gradual downstroke following peak amplitude, and usually the presence of a dicrotic notch. The first sign of possible abnormality is the absence of the dicrotic notch. More significant occlusions will show a decreased slope of the ascending and descending segments, and a rounding of the systolic peak occurs. More serious obstructions will show flattened waveforms. It is important to note that arteries located lower on the leg will produce sharper waveform peaks, while those located higher on the leg will produce more rounded waveforms.

11. Repeat for the other leg.

Instrumentation

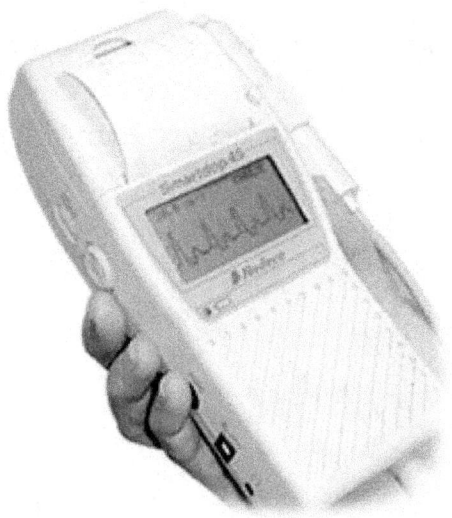

Smartdop® 45 Vascular Ultrasound Doppler

The Smartdop 45 vascular ultrasound doppler is recommended because it is portable, has a waveform LCD display, and a high resolution printer. Koven Technology, Inc. also provides training videos and a manual with the purchase of this doppler. It also has a button on the probe that allows the user to operate the instrument with only one hand.

Doppler Testing Equipment and Supplies

www.koven.com

Koven Technology, Inc.
12125 Woodcrest Executive Drive, Suite 320
St. Louis, MO 63141
Sales info: info@koven.com
800-521-8342

Smartdop 45 Vascular Ultrasound Doppler, $2,500.00

Accessories
VC-12 12 mm vascular cuff ($44)
VC-12 12 mm vascular cuff ($44)
VC-10 10mm vascular cuff ($44)
VC-10 10mm vascular cuff ($44)

Sphygmomanometer (SPG-1) ($85)

Doppler Printer Paper (PA-1) ($38)

Ultrasound Gel: 0102 Ultrasound Gel (box of 12 tubes) ($28.00)

Disinfectant Spray ($14.95)

from many vendors:

Kimberly-Clark Lavender Nitrile Powder-Free Exam Glove, KC100 latex free in various sizes

Measure your hand across the INSIDE PALM at the knuckles. Use the longest length or width to determine your correct glove size.

Items for Travel:

www.bestmasage.com

Best Massage 30" Echo BodyChoice Portable Massage Table, $129.00

www.ebags.com

A. Saks Ballistic Nylon Expandable Briefcase, $104

www.bhphotovideo.com

Tamrac MX5347 M.A.S. Lens Case (fits the Smartdop 45)

ABI Form

Lower Extremity Physiologic Study, Single Level (Ankle Brachial Index Assessment Form)

Patient's Name_____ ID#_____

Age_____ Date_____ Test Facility/Office_____

Risk Factors		Current Symptoms	ABI / Severity of Disease
☐ Tobacco Use	☐ Age over 50	☐ Intermittent Claudication	> 1.40 = Noncompressible
☐ Diabetes	☐ Hypertension	☐ Numbness, tingling in feet	1.00 - 1.40 = Normal
☐ Heart Disease	☐ Hyperlipemia	☐ Ulcerations	0.91 - 0.99 = Borderline
☐ Stroke/TIA	☐ Previous Vascular Surgery	☐ Other:	0.00 - 0.90 = Abnormal
☐ Overweight	☐ Impotence		2011 ACCF/AHA Guidelines
☐ High Fat Diet	☐ Family History Heart Disease	ICD:	
	☐ Other:		

Right Arm
Systolic Pressure _____ mmHg
☐ Triphasic (Normal)
☐ Biphasic (Diminished)
☐ Monophasic (Poor)

Left Arm
Systolic Pressure _____ mmHg
☐ Triphasic (Normal)
☐ Biphasic (Diminished)
☐ Monophasic (Poor)

Right ABI at Posterior Tibial
$$\frac{\text{Right PT Pressure}}{\text{Higher Arm Pressure}} = \underline{\quad\quad} = \underline{\quad\quad}$$

Right Posterior Tibial
Systolic Pressure _____ mmHg
☐ Triphasic (Normal)
☐ Biphasic (Diminished)
☐ Monophasic (Poor)

Left Posterior Tibial
Systolic Pressure _____ mmHg
☐ Triphasic (Normal)
☐ Biphasic (Diminished)
☐ Monophasic (Poor)

Right ABI at Dorsals Pedis
$$\frac{\text{Right DP Pressure}}{\text{Higher Arm Pressure}} = \underline{\quad\quad} = \underline{\quad\quad}$$

Left ABI at Posterior Tibial
$$\frac{\text{Right PT Pressure}}{\text{Higher Arm Pressure}} = \underline{\quad\quad} = \underline{\quad\quad}$$

Right Dorsalis Pedis
Systolic Pressure _____ mmHg
☐ Triphasic (Normal)
☐ Biphasic (Diminished)
☐ Monophasic (Poor)

Left Dorsalis Pedis
Systolic Pressure _____ mmHg
☐ Triphasic (Normal)
☐ Biphasic (Diminished)
☐ Monophasic (Poor)

Left ABI at Dorsalis Pedis
$$\frac{\text{Right DP Pressure}}{\text{Higher Arm Pressure}} = \underline{\quad\quad} = \underline{\quad\quad}$$

Right

☐ PT

☐ DP

Left

☐ PT

☐ DP

Insurance Reimbursement

Medicare insurance carriers impose varying degrees of restriction on who may be reimbursed for performing vascular examinations. Some carriers require only that the exam be performed by a person with adequate training and background. Other carriers recommend, but don't require, that the "studies either be rendered in a physician's office by/or under the direct supervision of persons credentialed in the specific type of procedure being performed or performed in laboratories accredited in the specific type of evaluation." The most restrictive Medicare carriers require that the exam be supervised by or performed by a physician, registered technician or specialist (RVT, RCVT, RVS), or by an accredited laboratory. The most recent Medicare reimbursement (2011) for the reimbursable ABI exam (CPT Code 93922) is an average of $114.

CPT Code: 93922 Non-invasive physiologic studies of upper or lower extremity arteries, single level, bilateral. Diagnostic (Medical Necessity) ICD9 codes for Procedure Code 93922:

250.70   Diabetes Mellitus with Peripheral Circulatory Disorders Type II or unspecified type not stated as uncontrolled
250.71   Diabetes Mellitus with Peripheral Circulatory Disorders Type I not stated as uncontrolled
250.72   Diabetes Mellitus with Peripheral Circulatory Disorders Type II or unspecified type uncontrolled
250.73   Diabetes Mellitus with Peripheral Circulatory Disorders Type I uncontrolled

353.00 Brachial plexus lesions

440.00 Atherosclerosis of aorta
440.20   Atherosclerosis of native arteries of the extremities unspecified
440.21   Atherosclerosis of native arteries of the extremities with intermittent claudication
440.22   Atherosclerosis of native arteries of the extremities with rest pain
440.23   Atherosclerosis of native arteries of the extremities with ulceration
440.24   Atherosclerosis of native arteries of the extremities with gangrene
440.30   Atherosclerosis of bypass graft of the extremities
440.31   Atherosclerosis of autologous vein bypass graft of the extremities
440.32   Atherosclerosis of nonautologous bilogical bypass graft of the extremities
441.00   Dissection of aorta aneruysm unspecified site
441.01   Dissection of aorta thoracic
441.02   Dissection of aorta abdominal
441.03   Dissection of aorta thoracoabdominal

441.10 Thoracic aneurysm, ruptured

441.20 Thoracic aneurysm without mention of rupture

441.30 Abdominal aneurysm, ruptured

441.40 Abdominal aneurysm without mention of rupture

441.50 Aortic aneurysm of unspecified site, ruptured

441.60 Thoracoabdominal aneurysm, ruptured

441.70 Thoracoabdominal aneurysm, without mention of rupture 441.90 Aortic aneurysm of unspecified site without mention of rupture

442.00 Aneurysm of artery of upper extremity 442.20 Other aneurysm, of iliac artery

442.30 Aneurysm of artery of lower extremity

443.00 Raynaud's syndrome

443.10 Thromboangiitis obliterans (Buerger's disease)

443.81 Peripheral angiopathy in diseases classified elsewhere

443.89   Other specified peripheral vascular diseases

443.90   Peripheral vascular disease, unspecified

444.00   Arterial embolism and thrombosis of abdominal aorta 444.10 Arterial embolism and thrombosis of thoracic aorta

444.21   Arterial embolism and thrombosis of the upper extremity

444.22   Arterial embolism and thrombosis of the lower extremity

444.81 Embolism and thrombosis of iliac artery

444.89   Embolism and thrombosis of other artery

444.90   Embolism and thrombosis of unspecified artery

447.00 Arteriovenous fistula, acquired 447.10 Stricture of artery

447.20 Rupture of artery

707.10   Ulcer of lower limbs, except decubitus

707.11   Ulcer of thigh

707.12   Ulcer of calf

707.13   Ulcer of ankle Continued on Back Page

707.14   Ulcer of heel and midfoot

707.15   Ulcer of other part of foot

707.80 Chronic ulcer of other specified sites

747.60 Anomaly of the peripheral vascular system, unspecified site

747.63   Upper limb vessel anomaly

747.64   Lower limb vesel anomaly

785.40 Gangrene

903.00   Injury to axillary vessel(s) unspecified

903.01   Injury to axillary artery

903.02   Injury to axillary vein

903.10 Injury to brachial blood vessels 903.20 Injury to radial blood vessels

903.30 Injury to ulnar blood vessels

903.40 Injury to palmar artery

903.50 Injury to digital blood vessels

903.80 Injury to other specified blood vessels of upper extremity 903.90 Injury to Unspecified blood vessel of upper extremity

904.00 Injury to femoral artery

904.10 Injury to superficial femoral artery 904.20 Injury to Femoral veins

904.30 Injury to Saphenous veins

904.40   Injury to Popliteal vessel(s) unspecified

904.41   Injury to popliteal artery

904.42   Injury to Popliteal vein

904.50   Injury to Tibial vessel(s), unspecified

904.51   Injury to anterior tibial artery

904.52   Injury to Anterior tibial vein

904.53   Injury to posterior tibial artery

904.54   Injury to posterior tibial vein

904.60 Injury to deep plantar blood vessels

904.70 Injury to other specified blood vessels of lower extremity 904.80 Injury to Unspecified blood vessel of lower extremity

904.90 Injury to blood vesels of lower extremity and unspecified sites

996.10 Mechanical complications of other vascular device, implant, and graft

996.70   Other complications due to unspecified device implant and graft

996.71   Other complications due to heart valve prosthesis

996.72   Other complications due to other cardiac device implant and graft

996.73   Other complications due to renal dialysis device implant and graft

996.74   Other complications due to other vascular device implant and graft

996.75   Other complications due to nervous system device implant and graft

996.76   Other complications due to genitourinary device implant and graft

996.77   Other complications due to internal joint prosthesis

996.78   Other complications due to other internal orthopedic device implant and graft

996.79   Other complications due to other internal prosthetic device implant and graft

998.11   Hemorrhage complicating a procedure

998.12   Hematoma complicating a procedure

998.13   Seroma complicating procedure

998.20 Atherosclerosis of native arteries of the extremities

V42.0 Organ or tissue replaced by transplant, Kidney

Nutrition for PAD

In this author's opinion, mild PAD is characterized as having an ABI between 0.91 and 1.4 and at least a biphasic Posterior Tibial waveform on one or both legs. It is in this early stage of PAD that nutrition and exercise may prevent further progression of PAD. In later stages it may also be helpful.

The following is nutritional information used in treating mild PAD and in general health. The nutritional information herein is intended to be an adjunct to medical treatment, not to replace medical treatment.

AVOID RED MEAT, ALCOHOL, SALT, CAFFEINE, AND TOBACCO.

DRINK MORE WATER.

IT IS IMPORTANT TO EXERCISE.

EAT A LOW FAT DIET.

Avoid cold remedies that contain pseudoephedrine (Advil Cold & Sinus, Aleve Sinus & Headache, Claritin-D, Sudafed, Tylenol Cold, Zyrtec-D, others) because they constrict your blood vessels.

Water

There is a great tendency for people to dehydrate from not drinking enough water. Drinking an adequate amount of water is probably the most important and the most ignored thing you can do for your body. Look at it this way. Seventy percent of your body is water. That's how important water is to your body. The mechanism the body uses for eliminating toxins is to convert them from fat-soluble to water-soluble so they can be excreted by the kidneys and skin. Drinking plenty of pure water will allow your body to rapidly excrete soluble waste products. Water is also important in moving material along the intestinal tract. Drink a minimum of 2 quarts of water per day. Drink a little more water than you think you need.

Water Calculator

Multiply weight in pounds by	0.5	_____
Multiply minutes of exercise per day by	0.1	_____
If pregnant, add	16	_____
If breast feeding, add	24	_____
If in a high altitude, add	8	_____
If in a dry climate, add	8	_____
Multiply number of caffeinated drinks per day by	4	_____
Multiply number of alcoholic drinks per day by	8	_____
If the weather very hot or very cold, add	16	_____
If there is fever or diarrhea, add	8	_____

Ounces of water needed per day – add totals	_____
Quarts of water needed per day – divide totals by 32	_____
8 oz. glasses of water needed per day – divide totals by 8	_____

Water Calculator References

Mayo Clinic
International Bottled Water Association
The United States Army Research Institute of Environmental Medicine
Center for Disease Control
Water for Good Health

Balancing Carbohydrates

A meal should have more carbohydrate than fat. If daily meals consists of more fat than carbohydrate, the brain will not have a sufficient amount of glucose, resulting in the production of ketones from fat for the brain to survive. This is a process called "ketosis," which can lead to other problems. A high fat diet will require a high amount of carbohydrates. Therefore, a diabetic should seek a low fat, low carbohydrate diet.

The American Diabetes Foundation recommends 45-60 g carbohydrates per meal for adults.

A meal should contain more carbohydrate calories than fat calories.

There is a carbohydrate balancing calculator in the library of www.allocca.com

Below are some balanced meal examples. An updated list can be found in the library of www.alloca.com

Food	Weight (g)	Fat (g)	Carbohydrate (g)	Protein (g)	Calories
Items for Meals					
Apple, raw, no skin, 1 medium	161.00	0.00	21.00	0.00	77.00
Banana, small, 6-7"	101.00	0.00	23.00	1.00	90.00
Butter, 1 pat, 1" square x 1/3" high	4.00	3.00	0.00	0.00	27.00
Cashew Flour 1 oz., 1/4 cup	28.00	14.00	8.00	5.00	160.00
Cashew nuts, raw 1/4 cup, 1 oz.	28.00	14.00	8.00	5.00	160.00
Cashew nut butter, 1 tablespoon	15.00	7.50	4.50	2.00	90.00
Chicken breasts - grilled	78.00	1.50	0.00	22.00	100.00
Chicken Curry	340.00	4.23	5.00	63.06	310.31
Coconut, raw, 1 oz.	28.00	9.00	4.00	1.00	99.00
Coconut, raw, 1 tablespoon	4.00	1.29	0.57	0.14	14.10
Corn, sweet, raw, 1 cup	154.00	2.00	29.00	5.00	132.00
Corn flakes or Puffs, lightly sweetened, 3/4 cup	30.00	0.00	27.00	2.00	110.00
Egg, 1 large	61.00	7.00	0.00	6.00	96.00
Granola, plain classic, Back to Nature brand, 1/2 cup	51.00	3.00	39.00	6.00	200.00
Ice Cream, Haagen-Dazs, Vanilla	92.00	15.00	18.00	4.00	220.00
Lentils, cooked, 1 cup	198.00	1.00	40.00	18.00	230.00
Oatmeal, Dry, 1/2 cup	40.00	3.00	26.00	6.00	155.00
Oatmeal, cooked, 1 cup	234.00	4.00	32.00	6.00	188.00
Olive Oil, 1 oz.	28.00	28.00	0.00	0.00	252.00
Olive Oil, 1 tablespoon	14.00	14.00	0.00	0.00	126.00
Potato, baked, 1	100.00	0.00	21.00	3.00	93.00
Potato, flakes, 1/3 cup	26.00	0.00	20.00	2.00	90.00
Potato, mashed with whole milk	210.00	1.00	37.00	4.00	210.00
Quinoa, cooked, 1 cup	185.00	4.00	39.00	8.00	224.00
Rice, Brown, 1 cup	195.00	2.00	46.00	5.00	218.00
Rice, white, California, 1 cup	186.00	0.00	53.00	4.00	242.00
Rice, Brown, Cake, Quaker, 1	9.00	0.00	7.00	1.00	35.00
Rice, Brown, Crispy Cereal, 1 cup	30.00	0.50	25.00	2.00	110.00
Rice, cracker, white, sesame, 1	1.75	0.13	1.38	0.13	6.88
Salad/Vegetables, 2 cups	72.00	0.00	2.00	0.00	8.00
Sesame Seeds, 1 cup	144.00	72.00	34.00	26.00	825.00
Strawberry, medium, 1	12.00	0.00	1.00	0.00	4.00
Sugar, granular, 1 packet	3.50	0.00	4.00	0.00	15.00
Sunflower Oil, 1 cup	218.00	218.00	0.00	0.00	1,927.00
Tomatoes, cooked, 1 cup	240.00	0.00	10.00	2.00	43.00
Tomato, raw, small, 1	91.00	0.00	4.00	1.00	16.00
Tomato Sauce, curry or Italian, with Olive Oil, 1 cup	247.00	7.00	10.00	2.00	106.00
Turkey (breast or dark meat)	170.00	2.80	7.20	29.00	176.00
Vegetable Curry	400.00	16.00	28.40	12.80	308.00

Food	Weight (g)	Fat (g)	Carbohydrate (g)	Protein (g)	Calories
Snack					
Cashew nuts, raw 1/2 cup (1 oz.)	56.00	28.00	16.00	10.00	320.00
Totals: Fat-70.79%, Carb-17.98%, Protein-11.24%	56.00	28.00	16.00	10.00	320.00
Snack					
Apple, raw, no skin, (1 medium)	161.00	0.00	21.00	0.00	77.00
Totals: Carb-100%	161.00	0.00	21.00	0.00	77.00
Snack					
Apple, raw, no skin, (1 medium)	161.00	0.00	21.00	0.00	77.00
Cashew Flour or Cashew nuts	23.80	11.90	6.80	4.25	151.30
Cold water	0.00	0.00	0.00	0.00	0.00
Totals: Fat-45.52%, Carb-47.26%, Protein-7.22%	184.80	11.90	27.80	4.25	235.30
Snack - Apple Cashew Dessert					
5 medium Apples, raw, no skin	805.00	0.00	105.00	0.00	385.00
1/2 cup Cashew nuts	69.51	34.76	19.86	12.42	441.90
1/2 cup Cashew flour	53.51	26.76	15.29	9.56	340.18
4 tablespoons unsweetened shredded coconut	16.00	5.16	2.28	0.56	56.40
4 Strawberries	48.00	0.00	4.00	0.00	16.00
1-1/4 cups water	0.00	0.00	0.00	0.00	0.00
Totals: Fat-47.04%, Carb-45.90%, Protein-7.07%	992.02	66.68	146.43	22.54	1,239.48
Divide recipe by 4			36.61		
Snack					
Granola, plain classic, Back to Nature brand	23.59	1.39	18.04	2.78	95.79
Cold water	0.00	0.00	0.00	0.00	0.00
Totals: Fat-13.06%, Carb-75.35%, Protein-11.59%	23.59	1.39	18.04	2.78	95.79
Snack					
Granola, plain classic, Back to Nature brand	39.23	2.31	30.00	4.62	159.27
Cold water	0.00	0.00	0.00	0.00	0.00
Totals: Fat-13.06%, Carb-75.35%, Protein-11.59%	39.23	2.31	30.00	4.62	159.27
Snack					
Granola, plain classic, Back to Nature brand	47.18	2.78	36.08	5.55	191.54
Cold water	0.00	0.00	0.00	0.00	0.00
Totals: Fat-13.06%, Carb-75.35%, Protein-11.59%	47.18	2.78	36.08	5.55	191.54

Food	Weight (g)	Fat (g)	Carbohydrate (g)	Protein (g)	Calories
Snack					
Rice, cracker, white, sesame, 1	1.75	0.13	1.38	0.13	6.88
10 Crackers	17.50	1.30	13.80	1.30	68.80
26 crackers	45.50	3.38	35.88	3.38	178.88
Totals: Fat-16.23%, Carb-76.56%, Protein-7.21%					
Snack					
Corn flakes, lightly sweetened	20.01	0.00	18.01	1.33	77.36
Cold water	0.00	0.00	0.00	0.00	0.00
Totals: Fat-0%, Carb-93.12%, Protein-6.88%	20.01	0.00	18.01	1.33	77.36
Snack					
Corn flakes, lightly sweetened	33.36	0.00	30.02	2.22	128.96
Cold water	0.00	0.00	0.00	0.00	0.00
Totals: Fat-0%, Carb-93.12%, Protein-6.88%	33.36	0.00	30.02	2.22	128.96
Snack					
Corn flakes, lightly sweetened	40.05	0.00	36.05	2.67	154.88
Cold water	0.00	0.00	0.00	0.00	0.00
Totals: Fat-0%, Carb-93.12%, Protein-6.88%	40.05	0.00	36.05	2.67	154.88
Snack					
Ice Cream, Haagen-Dazs, Vanilla	92.00	15.00	18.00	4.00	220.00
Totals: Fat-60.54%, Carb-32.29%, Protein-7.17%	184.00	30.00	36.00	8.00	446.00
Snack					
Rice, Brown, Cake, Quaker, 1	9.00	0.00	7.00	1.00	35.00
Totals: Fat-0%, Carb-87.50%, Protein-12.5%	9.00	0.00	7.00	1.00	35.00
Snack					
Rice, Brown, Cake, Quaker, 1	9.00	0.00	7.00	1.00	35.00
Butter, 1/4 pat	1.00	0.75	0.00	0.00	6.75
Totals: Fat-17.42%, Carb-72.26%, Protein-10.32%	10.00	0.75	7.00	1.00	41.75
Snack					
Banana, small, 6-7"	158.07	0.00	36.00	1.57	144.00
Totals: Fat-0%, Carb-95.82%, Protein-4.18%	158.07	0.00	36.00	1.57	144.00

Food	Weight (g)	Fat (g)	Carbohydrate (g)	Protein (g)	Calories
Breakfast					
Oatmeal, Dry	69.24	5.19	45.01	10.39	268.31
Hot water	0.00	0.00	0.00	0.00	0.00
Totals: Fat-17.41%, Carb-67.10%, Protein-15.49%	69.24	5.19	45.01	10.39	268.31
Breakfast					
Oatmeal, Dry	63.20	3.16	41.08	9.48	230.68
Sugar, granular, 1 packet	3.50	0.00	4.00	0.00	15.00
Hot water	0.00	0.00	0.00	0.00	0.00
Totals: Fat-11.53%, Carb-73.10%, Protein-15.37%	66.70	3.16	45.08	9.48	246.68
Breakfast					
Oatmeal, Dry	50.80	3.81	33.02	7.62	196.85
Sugar, granular, 1 packet	3.50	0.00	4.00	0.00	15.00
Hot water	0.00	0.00	0.00	0.00	0.00
Cashew Flour or Cashew nuts	28.00	14.00	8.00	5.00	178.00
Totals: Fat-41.01%, Carb-46.07%, Protein-12.92%	82.30	17.81	45.02	12.62	390.85
Breakfast					
Oatmeal, cooked	329.24	5.63	45.02	8.44	264.51
Totals: Fat-19.16%, Carb-68.08%, Protein-12.76%	329.24	5.63	45.02	8.44	264.51
Breakfast					
Oatmeal, cooked	300.23	5.13	41.06	7.70	241.21
Sugar, granular, 1 packet	3.50	0.00	4.00	0.00	15.00
Totals: Fat-17.95%, Carb-70.08%, Protein-11.97%	303.73	5.13	45.06	7.70	257.21
Breakfast					
Granola, plain classic, Back to Nature brand	58.91	3.47	45.05	6.93	239.15
Cold water	0.00	0.00	0.00	0.00	0.00
Totals: Fat-13.06%, Carb-75.35%, Protein-11.59%	58.91	3.47	45.05	6.93	239.15
Breakfast					
Granola, plain classic, Back to Nature brand	48.45	2.85	37.05	5.70	196.65
Cashew Flour or Cashew nuts	28.00	14.00	8.00	5.00	178.00
Cold water	0.00	0.00	0.00	0.00	0.00
Totals: Fat-40.08%, Carb-48.10%, Protein-11.42%	76.45	16.85	45.05	10.70	374.65

Food	Weight (g)	Fat (g)	Carbohydrate (g)	Protein (g)	Calories
Breakfast					
Corn flakes or Puffs, lightly sweetened	50.10	0.00	45.09	3.34	193.72
Cold water	0.00	0.00	0.00	0.00	0.00
Totals: Fat-0%, Carb-93.10%, Protein-6.9%	50.10	0.00	45.09	3.34	193.72
Breakfast					
Corn flakes or Puffs, lightly sweetened	41.13	0.00	37.02	2.74	159.04
Cashew Flour or Cashew nuts	28.00	14.00	8.00	5.00	178.00
Cold water	0.00	0.00	0.00	0.00	0.00
Totals: Fat-37.38%, Carb-53.43%, Protein-9.19%	69.13	14.00	45.02	7.74	337.04
Breakfast					
Rice, Brown, Crispy Cereal, 1 cup	54.00	0.90	45.00	3.60	202.50
Cold water	0.00	0.00	0.00	0.00	0.00
Totals: Fat-4%, Carb-88.90%, Protein-7.11%	54.00	0.90	45.00	3.60	202.50
Breakfast					
Rice, Brown, Crispy Cereal, 1 cup	44.40	0.74	37.00	2.96	166.50
Cashew Flour or Cashew nuts	28.00	14.00	8.00	5.00	178.00
Cold water	0.00	0.00	0.00	0.00	0.00
Totals: Fat-38.51%, Carb-52.25%, Protein-9.24%	72.40	14.74	45.00	7.96	344.50

Food	Weight (g)	Fat (g)	Carbohy drate (g)	Protein (g)	Calories
Lunch					
Chicken breasts - grilled (2) with white Rice	156.00	3.00	0.00	44.00	203.00
Rice, white, California	155.31	0.00	45.04	3.11	192.60
Olive Oil (1 tablespoon)	14.00	14.00	0.00	0.00	126.00
Totals: Fat-29.33%, Carb-34.54%, Protein-36.13%	325.30	17.00	45.04	47.11	421.60
Lunch					
Chicken breasts - grilled (2) with white Rice	156.00	3.00	0.00	44.00	203.00
Rice, brown	191.10	1.96	45.08	4.90	217.56
Olive Oil (1 tablespoon)	14.00	14.00	0.00	0.00	126.00
Totals: Fat-31.22%, Carb-32.99%, Protein-35.79%	361.10	18.96	45.08	48.80	546.56
Lunch					
Chicken breasts - grilled (2) with Potato	156.00	3.00	0.00	44.00	203.00
Potato, baked	214.50	0.00	45.05	6.44	205.96
Olive Oil (1 tablespoon)	14.00	14.00	0.00	0.00	126.00
Totals: Fat-28.6%, Carb-33.68%, Protein-37.71%	384.50	17.00	45.05	50.44	534.96
Lunch					
Chicken breasts - grilled (2) with Potato	156.00	3.00	0.00	44.00	203.00
Potato, flakes	58.50	0.00	45.00	4.50	198.00
Hot water	0.00	0.00	0.00	0.00	0.00
Olive Oil (1 tablespoon)	14.00	14.00	0.00	0.00	126.00
Totals: Fat-29.03%, Carb-34.16%, Protein-36.81%	228.50	17.00	45.00	48.50	527.00
Lunch					
Lentils, cooked	225.75	1.13	45.00	20.25	271.17
Totals: Fat-3.75%, Carb-66.38%, Protein-29.87%	225.75	1.13	45.00	20.25	271.17
Add on					
Corn, sweet, raw	239.00	3.11	45.04	7.77	239.23

Food	Weight (g)	Fat (g)	Carbohydrate (g)	Protein (g)	Calories
Dinner					
Chicken breasts - grilled (2) with white Rice & Salad	156.00	3.00	0.00	44.00	200.00
Rice, white, california	148.43	0.00	43.04	2.97	184.04
Salad/Vegetables 2 cups	72.00	0.00	2.00	0.00	8.00
Olive Oil (1 tablespoon)	14.00	14.00	0.00	0.00	126.00
Totals: Fat-29.36%, Carb-34.58%, Protein-36.06%	390.40	17.00	45.04	46.97	521.04
Dinner					
Chicken breasts - grilled (2) with white Rice & Salad	156.00	3.00	0.00	44.00	200.00
Rice, brown	182.33	1.87	43.01	4.68	207.59
Salad/Vegetables 2 cups	72.00	0.00	2.00	0.00	8.00
Olive Oil (1 tablespoon)	14.00	14.00	0.00	0.00	126.00
Totals: Fat-%, Carb-%, Protein-%	424.33	18.87	45.01	48.68	544.59
Dinner					
Chicken breasts - grilled (2) with Potato & Salad	156.00	3.00	0.00	44.00	200.00
Potato, baked	204.80	0.00	43.01	6.14	196.60
Salad/Vegetables 2 cups	72.00	0.00	2.00	0.00	8.00
Olive Oil (1 tablespoon)	14.00	14.00	0.00	0.00	126.00
Totals: Fat-28.67%, Carb-33.74%, Protein-37.59%	446.80	17.00	45.01	50.14	533.60
Dinner					
Chicken breasts - grilled (2) with Potato & Salad	156.00	3.00	0.00	44.00	200.00
Potato, flakes	55.90	0.00	43.00	4.30	189.20
Hot water	0.00	0.00	0.00	0.00	0.00
Salad/Vegetables 2 cups	72.00	0.00	2.00	0.00	8.00
Olive Oil (1 tablespoon)	14.00	14.00	0.00	0.00	126.00
Totals: Fat-29.08%, Carb-34.21%, Protein-36.72%	297.90	17.00	45.00	48.30	526.20
Dinner					
Chicken Curry (Indian Restaurant)	340.00	4.23	5.00	63.06	310.31
Rice, white	138.01	0.00	40.02	2.23	169.00
Totals: Fat-7.94%, Carb-37.57%, Protein-54.49%	478.01	4.23	45.02	65.29	479.31
Dinner					
Vegetable Curry (Indian Restaurant)	320.00	12.80	22.72	10.24	247.04
Rice, white	77.00	0.00	22.33	1.54	95.48
Totals: Fat-14.11%, Carb-80.71%, Protein-5.18%	397.00	12.80	45.05	11.78	342.52

Food	Weight (g)	Fat (g)	Carbohydrate (g)	Protein (g)	Calories
Dinner					
Chicken breast - grilled - Sweet Mama's Restaurant	174.00	3.35	0.00	49.06	226.39
Vegetables	345.60	0.00	9.60	0.00	48.00
Potato, baked	169.00	0.00	35.49	5.07	162.24
Totals: Fat-7.06%, Carb-42.24%, Protein-50.70%	688.60	3.35	45.09	54.13	427.03
Dinner					
Chicken breasts - grilled - Pumpernickel's Restaurant	160.00	3.08	0.00	45.14	208.28
Salad/Vegetables 2 cups	72.00	0.00	2.00	0.00	8.00
Mashed Potatoes with milk	244.44	1.16	43.07	4.66	201.36
Totals: Fat-9.14%, Carb-43.17%, Protein-47.70%	467.50	4.24	45.07	49.80	417.64
Dinner					
Turkey (breast or dark meat) with Brown Rice	170.00	2.80	7.20	29.00	170.00
Salad/Vegetables 2 cups	72.00	0.00	2.00	0.00	8.00
Rice, white, California	123.50	0.00	35.82	2.47	153.16
Olive Oil (1 tablespoon)	14.00	14.00	0.00	0.00	126.00
Totals: Fat-33.07%, Carb-39.39%, Protein-27.54%	379.50	16.80	45.02	31.47	457.16
Dinner					
Turkey (breast or dark meat) with Potato	170.00	2.80	7.20	29.00	170.00
Salad/Vegetables 2 cups	72.00	0.00	2.00	0.00	8.00
Potato, baked	170.50	0.00	35.81	5.12	163.72
Olive Oil (1 tablespoon)	14.00	14.00	0.00	0.00	126.00
Totals: Fat-32.33%, Carb-38.49%, Protein-29.18%	426.50	16.80	45.01	34.12	467.72
Dinner					
Turkey drumstick (456g total, 267 g meat) with Potato	267.00	4.40	11.30	45.53	266.92
Salad/Vegetables 2 cups	72.00	0.00	2.00	0.00	8.00
Potato, baked	151.00	0.00	31.71	4.53	144.96
Olive Oil (1 tablespoon)	14.00	14.00	0.00	0.00	126.00
Totals: Fat-30.34%, Carb-32.98%, Protein-36.68%	504.00	18.40	45.01	50.06	545.88
Add on					
Corn, sweet, raw	228.69	2.97	43.07	7.43	228.73

Food	Weight (g)	Fat (g)	Carbohydrate (g)	Protein (g)	Calories
A meal should have more carbohydrate than fat. If daily meals consists of more fat than carbohydrate, the brain will not have a sufficient amount of glucose, resulting in the production of ketones from fat for the brain to survive. This is a process called "ketosis," which can lead to other problems. A high fat diet will require a high amount of carbohydrates. Therefore, a diabetic should seek a low fat, low carbohydrate diet. A carbohydrate content of 45%-60% is recommended.					
The Gluten Test The first step is to measure blood glucose levels 2 hours after meals while avoiding all gluten products for 4 days. Re-introduce a gluten product, such as wheat, containing the same amount of carbohydrates, during a specific meal. Measure the blood glucose level after 2 hours. Compare the readings with and without gluten. Repeat this process several times. Blood glucose meters can be purchased at local pharmacies.					
The Dairy Test The first step is to measure blood glucose levels 2 hours after meals while avoiding all dairy products for 4 days. Re-introduce a dairy product, such as milk during a specific meal. Measure the blood glucose level after 2 hours. Compare the readings with and without dairy. Repeat this process several times. Blood glucose meters can be purchased at local pharmacies.					
American Diabetes Foundation recommends 45-60 grams carbohydrates per meal for adults					
A meal should contain more carbohydrate calories than fat calories.					
1 gram fat = 9 calories					
1 gram carbohydrate = 4 calories					
1 gram protein = 4 calories					
This chart provides the quantities of weight, fat, carbohydrate, protein, and calories for each meal. Each meal is designed to provide a adequate amount of balanced carbohydrate. A recommended scale is the American Weigh ONYX Slim Design Kitchen Scale. It is important to weigh the rice or potato for each meal.					

Dietary Rotation

Eating the same foods over and over again, can lead to a food sensitivity, whereby the body begins to react adversely to those foods. Approximately 90% of food sensitivities are acquired and 10% are inherited. Become aware of foods you are sensitive to, and eliminate them from your diet for at least one year. Symptoms of food sensitivity include: abdominal bloating, abdominal discomfort, skin rashes, fatigue increases after meals, headaches, body aches, swollen joints, alternating constipation and diarrhea, hyperactivity, nausea, etc. Milk is a very common allergy as well as intolerance. Food allergy cause allergic reactions throughout the body. Food intolerances cause indigestion or the lack of digestion of that particular food. Specific foods should not be consumed for more than four consecutive days.

Fresh, Whole, Living Food

Choose food that are certified organic and fresh. Regular food contain many pesticides and preservatives that are toxic to the body and known to be carcinogenic. Most processed and refined food contain ingredients that are toxic, carcinogenic, and chemically don't even resemble food. High fiber food are important for good intestinal health. Choose food that do not contain pesticides, saturated fats, red meats, additives, sugar, refined carbohydrates, excessive salt, alcohol, and caffeine. Avoid over-eating, which can lead to digestive problems and congestive bowel toxicity.

Caffeine

Caffeine has a detrimental effect on the body, especially the cardiovascular system. Caffeine may also mask your true energy level. Many people do not have enough energy to function without a substantial amount coffee every day. Caffeine is also addictive. The more caffeine you drink, the more caffeine your body will require for the same effect. If you are eating properly, and are in good health, you will not require the stimulation of caffeine to feel energetic.

A 5-ounce cup of coffee contains approximately 190 mg caffeine. A cup of tea varies from 10 to 90 mg. Regular use of more than 350 mg of caffeine per day causes physical dependence. 1 cup of coffee per day is not likely to cause addiction. Limit your intake coffee to not more than one cup per day and not more than 250 mg caffeine per day.

If your intake of caffeine is more than 250 mg per day, you will need to slowly withdraw from the caffeine addiction. For example, if you are consuming 6 cups of coffee per day, cut this down to 5 cups per day for 4 days, then 4 cups per day for 4 days, then 3 cups per day for 4 days, then 2 cups per day for 4 days, then 1 cup per day for 4 days. Do not exercise during this withdrawal period.

Caffeine Content of Foods and Drugs

Product	Serving Size	Caffeine (mg)
OTC Drugs		
NoDoz, maximum strength; Vivarin	1 tablet	200
Excedrin	2 tablets	130
NoDoz, regular strength	1 tablet	100
Anacin	2 tablets	64
Coffee		
Coffee, brewed	8 ounces	135
General Foods International Coffee, Orange Cappuccino	8 ounces	102
Coffee, instant	8 ounces	95
General Foods International Coffee, Cafe Vienna	8 ounces	90
Maxwell House Cappuccino, Mocha	8 ounces	60-65
General Foods International Coffee, Swiss Mocha	8 ounces	55
Maxwell House Cappuccino, French Vanilla or Irish Cream	8 ounces	45-50
House Cappuccino, Amaretto	8 ounces	25-30
General Foods International Coffee, Viennese Chocolate Café	8 ounces	26
Maxwell House Cappuccino, decaffeinated	8 ounces	3-6
Coffee, decaffeinated	8 ounces	5
Tea		
Celestial Seasonings Iced Lemon Ginseng Tea	16-oz. bottle	100
Bigelow Raspberry Royale Tea	8 ounces	83
Tea, leaf or bag	8 ounces	50
Snapple Iced Tea, all varieties	16-oz. bottle	42
Lipton Natural Brew Iced Tea Mix, unsweetened	8 ounces	25-45
Lipton Tea	8 ounces	35-40
Lipton Iced Tea, assorted varieties	16-oz. bottle	18-40
Lipton Natural Brew Iced Tea Mix, sweetened	8 ounces	15-35
Nestea Pure Sweetened Iced Tea	16-oz. bottle	34
Tea, green	8 ounces	30
Arizona Iced Tea, assorted varieties	16-oz. bottle	15-30
Lipton Soothing Moments Blackberry Tea	8 ounces	25

Product	Serving Size	Caffeine (mg)
Nestea Pure Lemon Sweetened Iced Tea	16-oz. bottle	22
Tea, instant	8 ounces	15
Lipton Natural Brew Iced Tea Mix, diet	8 ounces	10-15
Lipton Natural Brew Iced Tea Mix, Decaffeinated	8 ounces	< 5
Celestial Seasonings Herbal Tea, all varieties	8 ounces	0
Celestial Seasonings Herbal Iced Tea, bottled	16-oz. bottle	0
Lipton Soothing Moments Peppermint Tea	8 ounces	0

Soft Drinks

Product	Serving Size	Caffeine (mg)
Josta	12 ounces	58
Mountain Dew	12 ounces	55.5
Surge	12 ounces	52.5
Diet Coke	12 ounces	46.5
Coca-Cola Classic	12 ounces	34.5
Dr. Pepper, regular or diet	12 ounces	42
Sunkist Orange Soda	12 ounces	42
Pepsi-Cola	12 ounces	37.5
Barqs Root Beer	12 ounces	22.5
7-UP or Diet 7-UP	12 ounces	0
Barqs Diet Root Beer	12 ounces	0
Caffeine-free Coca-Cola or Diet Coke	12 ounces	0
Caffeine-free Pepsi or Diet Pepsi	12 ounces	0
Minute Maid Orange Soda	12 ounces	0
Mug Root Beer	12 ounces	0
Sprite or Diet Sprite	12 ounces	0

Caffeinated Waters

Product	Serving Size	Caffeine (mg)
Java Water (1/2 liter)	16.9 ounces	125
Krank 20 (1/2 liter)	16.9 ounces	100
Aqua Blast (1/2 liter)	16.9 ounces	90
Water Joe (1/2 liter)	16.9 ounces	60-70
Aqua Java (1/2 liter)	16.9 ounces	50-60

Frozen Desserts

Product	Serving Size	Caffeine (mg)
Ben & Jerry's No Fat Coffee Fudge Frozen Yogurt	1 cup	85
Starbucks Coffee Ice Cream, assorted flavors	1 cup	40-60
Häagen-Dazs Coffee Ice Cream	1 cup	58
Häagen-Dazs Coffee Frozen Yogurt, fat-free	1 cup	40

Product	Serving Size	Caffeine (mg)
Häagen-Dazs Coffee Fudge Ice Cream, low-fat	1 cup	30
Starbucks Frappuccino Bar	1 bar (2.5 oz.)	15
Healthy Choice Cappuccino Chocolate Chunk or Cappuccino Mocha Fudge Ice Cream…	1 cup	8

Yogurt, one container

Dannon Coffee Yogurt	8 ounces	45
Yoplait Cafe Au Lait Yogurt	6 ounces	5
Dannon Light Cappuccino Yogurt	8 ounces	< 1
Stonyfield Farm Cappuccino Yogurt	8 ounces	0

Chocolates or Candies

Hershey's Special Dark Chocolate Bar	1 bar (1.5 oz.)	31
Perugina Milk Chocolate Cappuccino Filling	1/3 bar (1.2 oz.)	24
Hershey Bar (milk chocolate)	1 bar (1.5 oz.)	10
Coffee Nips (hard candy)	2 pieces	6
Cocoa or Hot Chocolate	8 ounces	5

Low Glycemic Index Food

The endocrine system and the nervous system work together to regulate the appetite so that appropriate amounts of the appropriate foods are taken in. Refined white sugar has a high glycemic index and offsets this balance. This high-caloric dynamite explodes the pancreas and pituitary gland into hyper-secretion of hormones. Eating added sugar in various foods and drinks everyday chronically over-stimulates the pituitary and pancreas glands. The thyroid and adrenals also suffer. Many medical journals have implicated refined white sugar as a causative factor in: atherosclerosis, coronary heart disease, kidney disease, liver disease, shortening of life span, making blood platelets stick together, causing rise in serum triglycerides, and increasing the desire for coffee and tobacco.

Why is this important? When excess glucose enters the blood, excessive insulin is produced to transport the excess glucose to the fat cells for storage. Insulin increases the activity of a liver enzyme called HMG CoA reductase, which causes the liver to produce excessive cholesterol.

Cholesterol in the proper amount is necessary for many functions in the body, such as a major constituent of cell membranes, and hormones. Cholesterol becomes a problem only when there is an excess of it in the blood. This is why we want to avoid foods that have a high Glycemic Index.

Insulin increases the activity of an enzyme called delta 5 desaturase, which converts dihomogammalinolenic acid to arachidonic acid. Arachidonic acid produces vasoconstrictive and inflammatory eicosenoids, which lead to arteriosclerosis and cardiovascular disease. Arachidonic acid is also found in high levels in red meat and egg yolks.

Food that contain higher amounts of fiber, fat, and protein, will have a lower Glycemic Index. Fiber, fat, and protein slows the uptake of sugar into the blood stream. Foods that have a high glycemic index will be broken down into glucose faster and therefore enter the blood stream faster, hence causing more insulin to be produced.

The glycemic index is a relative scale for classifying foods according to the blood sugar response that they cause. It measures how fast the carbohydrate of a particular food is converted to glucose and enters the blood. The glycemic index for a particular food may be different for different individuals. The figures below contain the glycemic index values for the average individual.

The numbers used in the glycemic index are percentages with respect to a reference food. In this list, they are given with respect to glucose. For example, brown rice, which has a glycemic index of 58, raises blood sugar more than barley, which has a glycemic index of 26. A food is generally considered to have a high Glycemic Index if it is greater than 50 (1/2 of the value of glucose). Glycemic Index values of foods below are adjusted proportionately so that Glycemic Index of glucose is equal to 100.

The following list is a compilation of several Glycemic Index studies.

Bakery Products

Cake, sponge	48
Cake, banana, made with sugar	49

Cake, pound	56
Pizza, cheese	63
Muffins	64
Cake, flan	68
Cake, angel food	69
Croissant	70
Crumpet	72
Donut	79
Waffles	80

Beverages

Coffee and Tea	0
Soy milk	31

Soft drink, Fanta	71
Rice milk	85
Lucozade	99

Bread

Bürgen Soy Lin	20
Bürgen Oat Bran & Honey Loaf	31
Barley kernel bread	40
Rye Kernel bread	48
Fruit loaf	49
Oat bran bread	50
Mixed grain bread	50

Pumpernickel	52
Bulger bread	55
Linseed rye bread	57
Pita bread, white	60
Whole grain bread	65
Rye flour bread	67
Semolina bread	67
Oat kernel bread	68

Barley flour bread	69
Wheat bread, wholemeal flour	72
Melba toast	73
Wheat bread, white	74
Bagel, white	75
Wheat bread, gluten free	94
French baguette	99

Breakfast Cereals

Rice Bran	20
All-bran	44

Bran Buds	55
Special K	56
Oat Bran	57
Muesli	58
Porridge (oatmeal)	64
Nutri-grain	69
Grapenuts	70
Shredded Wheat	72
Cream of Wheat	73
Puffed Wheat	77
Cheerios	77
Corn Bran	78
Total	80
Cocopops	80
Rice Krispies	85
Cornflakes	87
Crispix	91
Rice Chex	93

Cereal Grains

Bran, wheat or oat	15
Wheat germ	15
Barley, pearled	26
Rye	35
Kamut (heat)	40
Oats	40
Wheat kernels	43

Bulgur	50	Yogurt, low fat, artificially sweet	15
Rice, parboiled	50	Milk	30
----		Yogurt, low fat, fruit sugar sweet	34
Barley, cracked	53	Milk, chocolate, sugar sweetened	36
Wheat, quick cooking	56	----	
Buckwheat	57	Ice Cream	64
Sweet corn	57		
Rice, brown	58		
Rice, wild, Saskatchewan	59	**Flours**	
Oatmeal	60	Almond Flour	15
Pearled Barley	60	Cashew Flour	15
Rice, white	61	Soy Flour	25
Barley, rolled	69	Rye Flour	45
Taco shells	71	Quinoa Flour	45
Cornmeal	72	Kamut Flour	45
Millet	74	----	
Tapioca, boiled with milk	84	Chestnut Flour	65
Puffed rice	85	Potato Starch	95
Rice, instant, boiled 6 min.	93	White Rice Flour	95
		Arrow Root Starch	85
		White Wheat Flour	85
Cookies		Whole wheat flour	80

Oatmeal	58		
Rich Tea	58		
Shortbread	66		
Arrowroot	69	**Fruit**	
Graham	77	Cherries	23
Vanilla	80	Raspberries, fresh	25
		Strawberries	25
		Grapefruit	30
Crackers		Apricots, dried	32
----		Apple	35
High Fibre Rye Crispread	68	Coconut	35
Breton Wheat Crackers	70	Oranges	35
Stoned Wheat Thins	70	Peaches	35
Water Crackers	74	Plums	35
Rice Cakes	80	Coconut Milk	40
Puffed Crispbread	85	Pear, fresh	39
		Plum	40
Dairy Foods		Apple juice	42
Cream	0	Peach, fresh	44

Pineapple, fresh	45	**Nuts/Seeds**	
Orange	46	Almonds	15
Grapes	45	Hazel nuts	15
Pineapple juice	48	Cashew nuts	15
Grapefruit juice	50	Walnuts	15
----		Sunflower seeds	35
Orange juice	54	Chestnut	60
Kiwifruit	55		
Mango	58	**Pasta**	
Apricots, fresh	60	Spaghetti, protein enriched	28
Banana	60	Fettuccine	34
Raisins	66	Vermicelli	37
Muskmelon or Cantaloupe	68	Star pastina	39
Pineapple	69	Spaghetti, white	43
Watermelon	75	Linguine	47
		Instant noodles	49
Legumes		Whole wheat	50
Soy beans, canned	15	----	
Soy beans	18	Spaghetti, durum	57
Lentils, red	26	Lasagna (hard wheat)	60
Beans, dried	29	Couscous	68
Lentils	30	Gnocchi	69
White beans	35	Lasagna (soft wheat)	75
Kidney beans	40	Rice pasta, brown	96
Split peas, yellow, boiled	33		
Lima beans, baby, frozen	34	**Rice**	
Garbanzo beans	34	Wild rice	35
Navy beans	39	Brown basmati rice	45
Pinto beans	40	Basmati rice	50
Black-eyed beans	43	Brown rice	50
Garbanzo beans, canned	44	----	
Pinto beans, canned	47	White rice	72
Romano beans	47		
Baked beans, canned	50	**Root Vegetables**	
----		Onions	15
Kidney beans, canned	54	Garlic	30
Lentils, green, canned	54	----	
Kidney beans, canned	54	Carrots	51
Beans, dried, P. vulgaris	73	Yam	53
Broad beans (fava beans)	82	Sweet potato	56

Beets	66
Potato, steamed	68
Rutabaga	75
Potato, boiled, mashed	76
French fries	78
Potato, instant	86
Potato, baked	88
Potato, fried	95
Parsnips	101

Snack Food

Peanuts	15
Peanut button, unsweetened	40

Jams and marmalades	51
Chocolate	51
Potato crisps	56
Popcorn	58
Mars Bar	66
Life Savers	73
Corn chips	77
Jelly beans	83
Pretzels	85
Dates	103

Soup

Tomato Soup	39
Lentil soup, canned	46

Split pea soup	63
Black bean soup	67
Green pea soup, canned	69

Sugars/Sweeteners

Stevia	0
Fructose (twice as sweet as sucrose)	23
Lactose	47

Honey	61
High fructose corn syrup	65
Maple Syrup	65
Sucrose	67
Glucose	100
Maltodextrin	110
Maltose	110
Corn Syrup	115

Vegetables

Celery	15
Fennel	15
Mushrooms	15
Olives	15
Lettuce	15
Spinach	15
Sprouted seeds	15
Eggplant	20
Peas, dried	23
Tomatoes	30
Turnip, raw	30
Peas, green	35
Marrowfat, dried	41
Peas, green	50

Sweet corn	65
Pumpkin	78
Turnip, cooked	85

References

Frati-Munari, A.C. , The Glycemic Index of Some Foods Common in Mexico, Gac Med Mex, Vol. 127, No. 2, March-April 1991

Jenkins, David J.A. et al., Glycemic Index of Foods: a Physiological Basis for Carbohydrate Exchange; (The American Journal of Clinical

Jenkins, D.J.A. and Jenkins, A.L. Treatment of hypertriglceridemia and diabetes; (Journal of the American College of Nutrition.

Jenkins, David J.A. et al., Starchy Foods and Glycemic Index; Diabetes Care, Vol. 11, No. 2, February 1988.

Miller, Janette Brand, et al, Rice: a High or Low Glycemic Index Food?; The American Journal of Clinical Nutrition, Vol. 56, 1992.

Miller, Janette C. Brand., Importance of Glycemic Index in Diabetes; The American Journal of Clinical Nutrition, Vol. 59 (supplement), 1994.

Miller, Janette Brand, International tables of glycemic index; The American Journal of Clinical Nutrition, Vol. 62 (supplement), 1995.

Rassmussen, Ole., Day-to-day Variation of the Glycemic Response in Subjects with Insulin-dependent Diabetes with Standardized Premeal Blood Glucose and Prandial Insulin Concentrations; The American Journal of Clinical Nutrition, Vol. 57, 1993.

Smith, Ulf., Carbohydrates, Fat, and Insulin Action; The American Journal of Clinical Nutrition, Vol. 59 (supplement), 1994

Wolever, Thomas M.S. et al., The Glycemic Index: Methodology and Clinical Implications The American Journal of Clinical Nutrition, Vol. 54, 1991.

Wolever, Thomas M.S. et al., Glycemic Index of Fruits and Fruit Products in Patients with Diabetes; The International Journal of Food Sciences and Nutrition, Vol. 43, 1993.

www.montignac.com

Eicosanoids

Eicosanoid is pronounced "eye-cos-san-oid." Eicosanoids are chemical messengers that are classified as two different types, pro-inflammatory and anti-inflammatory. The pro-inflammatory variety stimulate vasoconstriction, platelet aggregation, tissue repair, clot formation, allergic responses, renin secretion, increased glycogenolysis, immune suppression, insulin release inhibition, and norepinephrine release inhibition. So, what's wrong with all of that? Clotting is good when you have a cut or injury, but not good in small blood vessels under normal conditions. Vasoconstriction is good when your blood pressure falls, but not good when your blood pressure is high. Inflammation is good when you have an injury or infection, but not good under normal conditions. Allergic responses are good when there is something in the environment that is toxic, but not when it is out of control. There's more, but I think you've gotten the message. You want to produce the anti-inflammatory eicosanoids when the body is normal and the pro-inflammatory eicosanoids only when there is a need for them.

How can we control eicosanoids? Our diet directly affects which eicosanoids are produced. To understand this, we need to look further into eicosanoid pathways. Let's start with Lineolic Acid. Lineolic Acid is an essential fatty acid that is contained in seed and vegetable oils, legume's, and mother's milk. With the appropriate enzymes, it can be either converted into other fatty acids that produce anti-inflammatory eicosanoids, such as series 1 Prostaglandins, or into a fatty acid such as, arachidonic acid that produce the pro-inflammatory eicosanoids, such as the series 2 prostaglandins, thromboxanes, and leukotrienes. Leukotrienes are 1,000 times more inflammatory than Prostaglandins and 1,000 to 10,000 times more inflammatory than histamine. Arachidonic acid is found in abundance in animal products, especially red meat.

Eicosapentanoic Acid (EPA) and Docosahexanoic Acid (DHA) produce anti-inflammatory eicosanoids such as, the series 3 Prostaglandins. This is a good thing. EPA and DHA also displaces arachidonic acid, reduces demand for cholesterol synthesis, stimulates metabolism of fat stores, activates T lymphocytes, and enhances action of insulin. This is a very good thing. EPA and DHA are commonly referred to as the Omega 3 fatty acids or "marine lipids." Fish, salmon in particular, are rich in EPA and DHA. EPA and DHA are also found in mother's milk and some seed oils. If you take an EPA/DHA supplement you want to be sure that the source is not from fish caught in polluted waters.

If you want to relieve pain and inflammation such as in arthritis, you may take an aspirin or other NSAID to block the inflammatory eicosanoid pathway. However, NSAID's block all of the pathways, pro-inflammatory and anti-inflammatory. Blocking the anti-inflammatory eicosanoids can weaken the immune system, degrade nerve function, etc. NSAID's may not be the best approach to pain.

What does this have to do with diet? Fatty acids are all available in our diet. Arachidonic Acid comes from animal products, mostly red meat. So, we want to limit our consumption of red meat as much as possible. Also, the enzyme that stimulates the production of Arachidonic acid is stimulated by insulin. Eating foods high in sugar will stimulate an insulin response and hence stimulate the production of Arachidonic Acid and pro-inflammatory eicosanoids.

The next time you eat, think first. Think about the consequences of what you're eating and how it will react in your body.

Omega 6 Fatty Acid - Eicosanoid Pathways

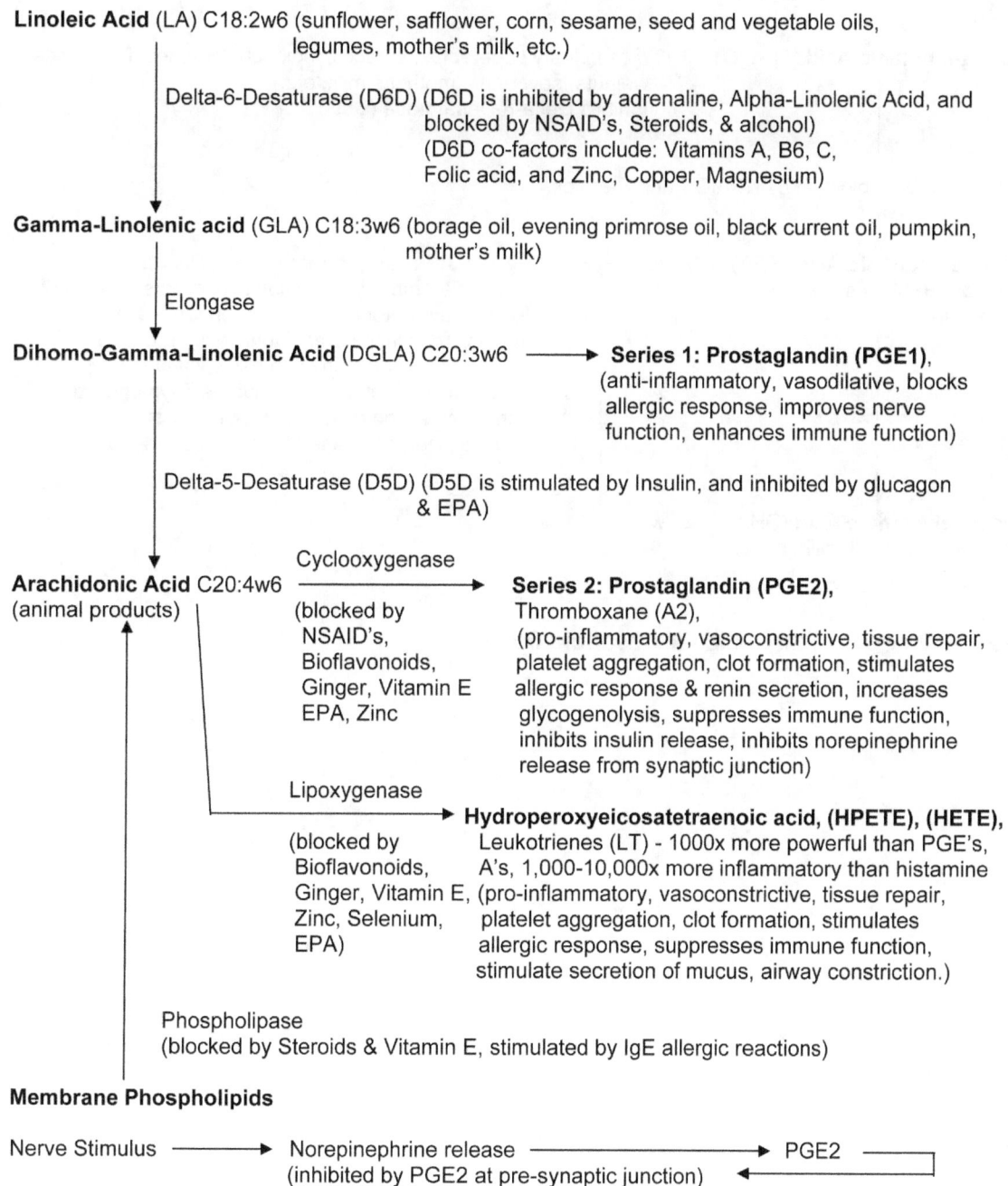

Linoleic Acid (LA) C18:2w6 (sunflower, safflower, corn, sesame, seed and vegetable oils, legumes, mother's milk, etc.)

Delta-6-Desaturase (D6D) (D6D is inhibited by adrenaline, Alpha-Linolenic Acid, and blocked by NSAID's, Steroids, & alcohol)
(D6D co-factors include: Vitamins A, B6, C, Folic acid, and Zinc, Copper, Magnesium)

Gamma-Linolenic acid (GLA) C18:3w6 (borage oil, evening primrose oil, black current oil, pumpkin, mother's milk)

Elongase

Dihomo-Gamma-Linolenic Acid (DGLA) C20:3w6 ⟶ **Series 1: Prostaglandin (PGE1)**,
(anti-inflammatory, vasodilative, blocks allergic response, improves nerve function, enhances immune function)

Delta-5-Desaturase (D5D) (D5D is stimulated by Insulin, and inhibited by glucagon & EPA)

Cyclooxygenase

Arachidonic Acid C20:4w6 ⟶ **Series 2: Prostaglandin (PGE2)**,
(animal products)   Thromboxane (A2),
(blocked by   (pro-inflammatory, vasoconstrictive, tissue repair,
NSAID's,   platelet aggregation, clot formation, stimulates
Bioflavonoids,   allergic response & renin secretion, increases
Ginger, Vitamin E   glycogenolysis, suppresses immune function,
EPA, Zinc   inhibits insulin release, inhibits norepinephrine
                       release from synaptic junction)

Lipoxygenase

⟶ **Hydroperoxyeicosatetraenoic acid, (HPETE), (HETE)**,
(blocked by   Leukotrienes (LT) - 1000x more powerful than PGE's,
Bioflavonoids,   A's, 1,000-10,000x more inflammatory than histamine
Ginger, Vitamin E,   (pro-inflammatory, vasoconstrictive, tissue repair,
Zinc, Selenium,   platelet aggregation, clot formation, stimulates
EPA)   allergic response, suppresses immune function,
                       stimulate secretion of mucus, airway constriction.)

Phospholipase
(blocked by Steroids & Vitamin E, stimulated by IgE allergic reactions)

Membrane Phospholipids

Nerve Stimulus ⟶ Norepinephrine release ⟶ PGE2
                (inhibited by PGE2 at pre-synaptic junction)

Figure 1 illustrates the Omega 6 Eicosanoid pathway. Figure 2 illustrates the Omega 3 Eicosanoid pathways.

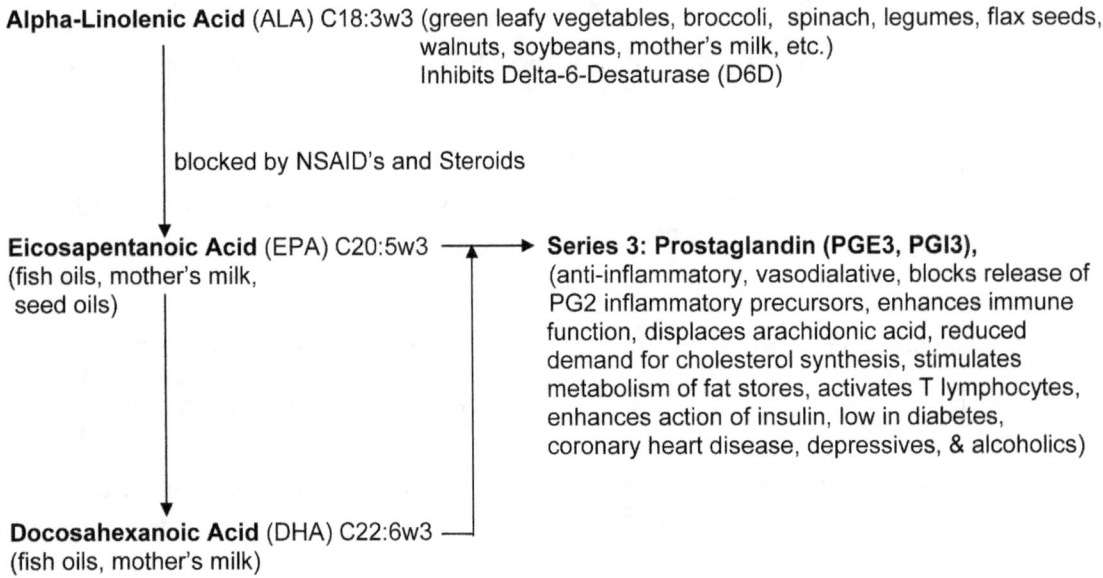

Figure 2 – Omega 3 Fatty Acid – Eicosanoid Pathways

Detoxification

Damage to the cells from toxins is the major cause of many health problems. Detoxifying and ridding the body of toxins, particularly neurotoxins, which deplete serotonin and norepinephrine, is an important part of balancing serotonin and norepinephrine levels.

Toxicity from foreign chemicals (exotoxins) can cause damage to almost all cells of the body. Symptoms include: fatigue, headaches, neurological disorders, chemical sensitivities, immune dysfunction, and liver disorders. Food is often the main source of toxins. There are thousands of chemicals used by the food industry during processing and packaging. Many farmers use pesticides on their produce, which are passed to consumers. In addition to these external sources of toxins, the body also produces toxins internally called, endotoxins resulting from digestion, immune system functions, emotional stress, etc. Endotoxins may also be produced as the result of food allergies and sensitivities.

Fat-soluble toxins are easily absorbed but poorly excreted. Often, they accumulate in the body causing damage to the tissues and organs, and depleting serotonin and norepinephrine. Fat-soluble chemicals are converted to water-soluble chemicals, primarily in the liver, and in some cells, in a two-step process so that the water-soluble toxins can be excreted by the urine, liver, and skin. The skin is a vitally important organ that eliminates toxins through perspiration.

During the first phase of detoxification, fat-soluble chemicals are converted into intermediate chemicals. As a result of this process, free radicals are produced. The free radicals and the intermediate chemicals can cause damage to the cells. An adequate amount of antioxidants must be present to detoxify these intermediate compounds produced during the first phase of detoxification. The first phase may also detoxify some chemicals directly without requiring a second phase conversion.

During the second phase, the intermediate chemicals are converted into water-soluble, chemicals, which are less toxic and easily excreted in the urine, bile, and skin.

It is very important to avoid toxic chemicals from the environment. Tap water should be filtered to remove lead, chlorine, heavy metals, and bacteria. It is also important to consume an adequate supply of anti-oxidants to prevention cellular damage.

The ability of the liver to detoxify is determined by the availability of the appropriate nutrients and enzymes. An adequate supply of antioxidants is vitally important after the first phase of converting fat-soluble toxins, which produce free radicals. Reduced glutathione, superoxide dismutase, and catalase are the primary antioxidants used in the body to neutralize free radicals. Other antioxidants include: beta-carotene, vitamin E, vitamin C, selenium, nacetylcysteine, lipoic acid, and proanthocyanidins. Vitamin and mineral cofactors required for cytochrome P-450 reactions include: riboflavin, niacin, magnesium, iron, and other trace minerals. Phytochemicals such as indoles from cruciferous vegetables and quercetin also help during the first phase of detoxification. Other second phase conjugating agents include amino acids such as glycine, cysteine, glutamine, methionine, taurine, glutamic acid, and asparatic acid.

Vitamin, mineral, and protein deficiencies will decrease the activity of the detoxification pathways. Fats and polyunsaturated oils can promote the uptake of many chemical carcinogens in the gastrointestinal tract. Olive oil (monounsaturated) and omega 3 polyunsaturated oils (EPA, DHA) have a neutral effect in promoting the uptake of carcinogens in the gastrointestinal tract.

As previously discussed, the detoxification process requires various nutrients to function. Without such nutrients in the cells, intermediate compounds can cause cellular and DNA damage. If the apoptosis system (cells self destruct if they are damaged) does not get the proper nutrients, the damaged cells can reproduce. If the immune system does not get the proper nutrients, the damaged cells can reproduce out of control causing cancer.

Transporting the nutrients into the blood is only the first step. The nutrients must enter the cells in order to be available for use by the cells. In order for the nutrients to get into the cells, they must be transported though the cell membrane. When there is a lack of nutrients, particularly oxygen inside the cell, there is a build-up of lactic acid inside the cell. Excessive lactic acid damages the cell membrane transport mechanism and DNA. Lactic acid causes the cell to become acidic (lower pH). There is a correlation between intracellular pH and urine pH. The urine pH must be 6.5 or greater, which indicates the maximum amount of lactic acid in the cell, for the membrane transport mechanisms to function at peak performance.

The detoxification process requires various nutrients to function properly. Without such nutrients in the cells, intermediate compounds can cause cellular and DNA damage. If the apoptosis system (cells self destruct if they are damaged), does not get the proper nutrients, the damaged cells can reproduce. If the immune system does not get the proper nutrients, the damaged cells can reproduce out of control causing cancer.

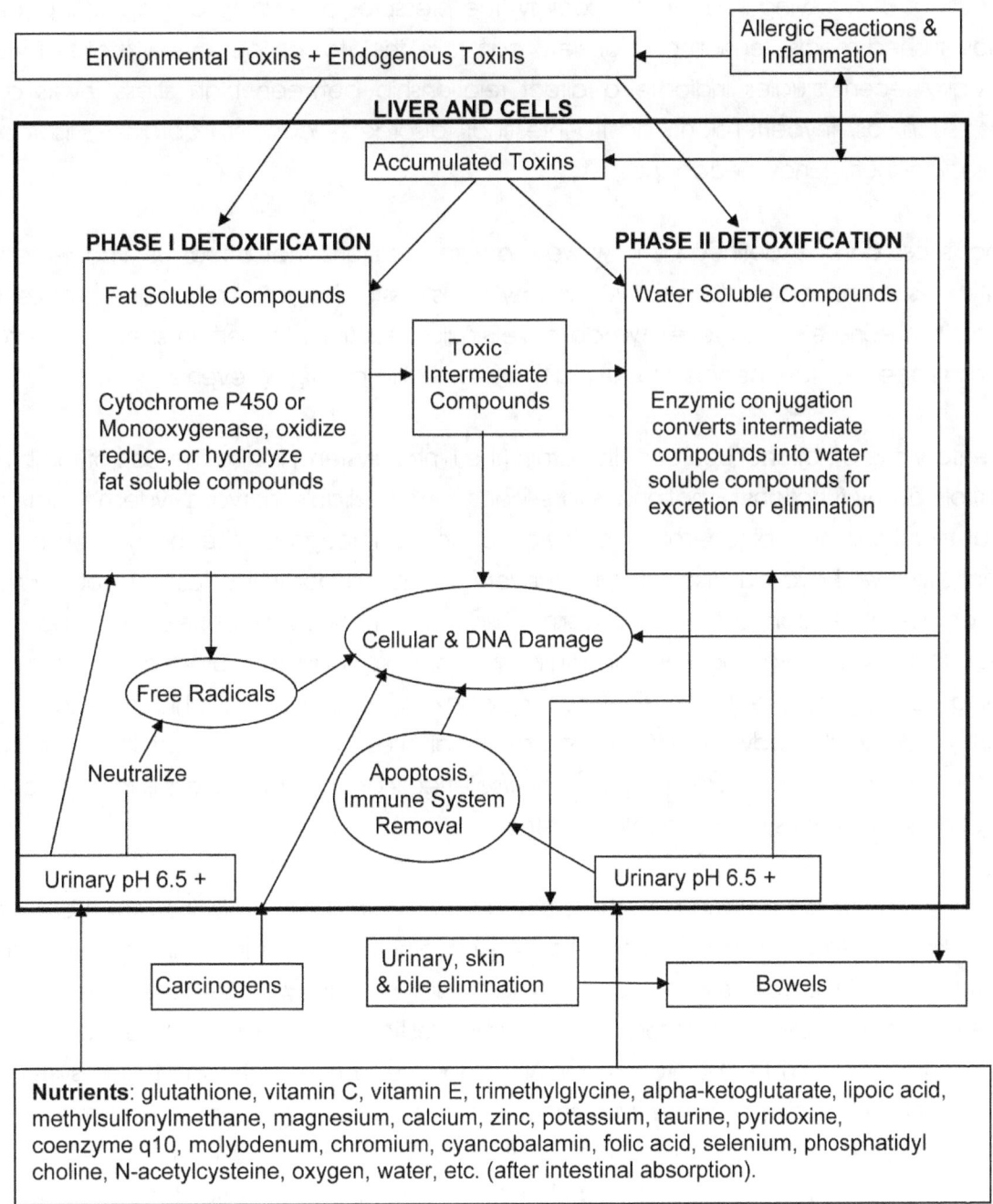

Figure 3 - Detoxification Pathways

The Physiological Effects of Emotional Stress

Today, most of us are living in a stressful society. The pressures of earning a living, fast paced schedules, rushed meals, tension and anxiety, can take their toll on our overall state of well-being. Many recent studies indicate a direct relationship between high stress levels and diseases such as, hypertension, gastro-intestinal disorders, cancer, cardiac disorders, immunological inefficiency, headaches, etc.

Emotional stress can be defined as how we react to situations that affect us. People react differently to specific circumstances. What may be stressful for you, may not be quite as stressful for someone else. However, we do have similar reactions to certain specific stresses, such as marriage, divorce, personal loss, and many other life-changing events.

Coincidentally, the emotional center of the brain (the limbic system) is also the part of the brain that controls bodily functions. Emotional stress leads to undesirable nervous system reactions, hormonal reactions and biochemical pathway changes throughout the body. Continuous emotional stress will have adverse effects on every cell in the body. It does not appear that nutrition or medicine can adequately compensate for the adverse effects of long-term hormonal, leukotriene, thromboxane, and inflammatory prostaglandin production. However, consuming foods that are high in Glycemic Index and high in arachidonic acid, will significantly add to the adverse effects of emotional stress. It appears that the best and possibly the only method for eliminating the adverse effects of emotional stress is to reduce the emotional stress by various stress reduction methods.

The limbic system consists of the hypothalamus and the surrounding regions of the cerebral cortex, working together as a whole system. The hypothalamus controls all the autonomic nervous functions of the body such as, body temperature, osmolality of the body, thirst, hunger, body weight, heart rate, respiratory rate, gastrointestinal functions, etc. Basically, the hypothalamus controls all the bodily functions that don't require thought. The limbic system is also the center of emotions, where emotional memories are stored. Emotions have direct pathways that effect bodily functions through the limbic system. One common emotional reaction that stimulates a physiological reaction is sadness, which stimulates the production of tears. The limbic system is also active in receiving and processing sensory signals for pain or pleasure.

Throughout the entire brain stem, there are areas of diffuse, short axon neurons that make multiple connections, known as the reticular formation or the reticular activating system. This system can be viewed as a kind of switching station that directs signals between the cerebrum and the autonomic nervous system.

The autonomic nervous system consists of the sympathetic nervous system and the parasympathetic nervous system. Sympathetic nervous stimulation dilates the pupils, increases heart rate and contractile force, constricts systemic blood vessels, increases blood coagulation and glucose, increases adrenal cortical secretion, increases mental activity, decreases kidney output, decreases peristalsis of the gut, increases strength and glycogenolysis of the skeletal muscles, etc. Glycogenolysis is the break down of glycogen to re-form glucose. The parasympathetic system effectively has the opposite effects on the same organs. The parasympathetic nervous system functions mainly to inhibit the sympathetic nervous system in a negative feedback loop. The activity of the autonomic nervous system can be controlled by the hypothalamus and the cerebrum. Many behavioral responses are effected by areas of the cerebrum sending signals to the hypothalamus, which sends signals through the reticular formation to the autonomic nervous system. The cerebrum can affect the entire autonomic nervous system severely enough to cause autonomic-induced disease such as gastric ulcers, constipation, heart palpitation, and heart attacks.

Excessive sympathetic stimulation may propagate a long-term hormonal effect on the body. For example, excessive sympathetic stimulation causes the adrenal medullae to produce large quantities of epinephrine (adrenaline) and norepinephrine. Normally, the ratio is 80% epinephrine and 20% norepinephrine. Epinephrine has almost the same effects as sympathetic stimulation. However, the epinephrine effects last about 10 times longer than the short-term sympathetic effects. Epinephrine has a stronger effect on cardiac activity, metabolism, increased metabolic activities such as, glycogenolysis in the liver and muscle, and glucose release into the blood than norepinephrine. Norepinephrine has a stronger vasoconstrictive effect on the blood vessels than epinephrine. Both epinephrine and norepinephrine increase the activity of the heart, inhibit peristalsis in the gastrointestinal tract, dilate the pupils, etc.

Anxiety is an emotional reaction that causes sympathetic stimulation by the cerebrum stimulating the hypothalamus and the autonomic nervous system through the reticular activating system. Environmental stimulation such as traffic, loud noises, ordinary fluorescent lighting, computer cathode ray tube monitors, and many others, can constantly stimulate our sympathetic nervous systems. Ordinary fluorescent lighting and cathode ray tube monitors and televisions, cause a flicker at 30 and 60 hertz, which cannot be detected by the human eye. However, this flicker can be detected by the brain causing the brain to become stimulated constantly by the flicker. Compact fluorescent bulbs with an electronic ballast (usually have a regular light bulb base), do not flicker and have a full spectrum of colors. Full spectrum of colors in lighting has a similar effect on us as daylight. Liquid crystal display computer monitors, which are also used in laptop computers, do not have a 30 or 60 hertz flicker.

If your daily stress level is high, you should look into stress reduction methods such as yoga, meditation, spirituality, psychotherapy, E.M.D.R., relaxation techniques and devices, etc.

Nervous System Stress Pathways

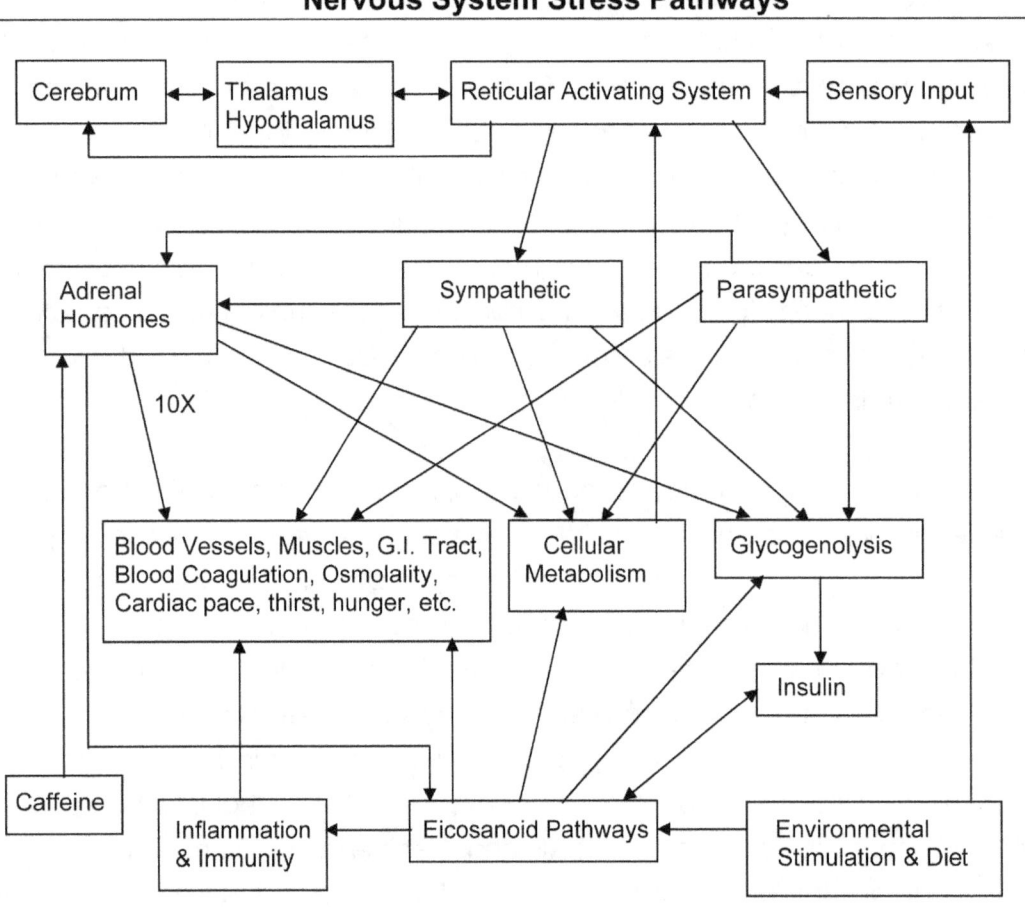

Figure 4 - Nervous System and Hormonal Pathways

Carbohydrate Craving

Serotonin

Serotonin (5-hydroxytryptamine, or 5-HT) is a neurotransmitter. Serotonin cannot cross the blood-brain barrier and therefore, must be produced within the brain. About 90 percent of serotonin is produced in the gastrointestinal tract.

Low serotonin levels in the brain are associated with migraine headaches, depression, insomnia, bipolar syndrome, increased anger and outbursts, increased aggression, bipolar disorder, anxiety disorder, increased body temperature, moody and socially withdrawn, decreased sexuality, increased appetite for carbohydrates, irritable bowel syndrome, tinnitus, fibromyalgia, increased escape fantasies and need for change, premenstrual syndrome (PMS), and seasonal affective disorder (SAD).

Some drugs inhibit the re-uptake of serotonin making it stay in the synapse longer.

"Long-term, but not short-term, antidepressant treatment decreases the numbers of both serotonin and beta-adrenergic receptors. The decrease in the number of receptor sites is most marked for [3H] spiroperidol-labeled serotonin receptors and is characteristic for antidepressants of several classes[2]."

Serotonin is manufactured from the amino acid tryptophan. Tryptophan is the least abundant essential amino acid. An essential amino acid cannot be produced by the body and must be included in the diet. It requires an albumin carrier to cross the blood-brain. 5-Hydroxytryptophan is the second step in serotonin production that does not require an albumin carrier to transport into the brain. 5-Hydroxytryptophan is more effective in producing serotonin than is tryptophan because it is a metabolite of tryptophan. Common food sources of tryptophan are bananas, dried dates, milk, yogurt, cottage cheese, red meat, eggs, fish, poultry, sesame, chickpeas, sunflower seeds, pumpkin seeds, and peanuts[4].

Norepinephrine

Norepinephrine is a hormone in the blood and a neurotransmitter in the central nervous system. Norepinephrine is related to attention and responding actions. Along with epinephrine, norepinephrine plays an important role in the fight-or-flight response, increasing heart rate, triggering the release of glucose from energy stores, increasing wakefulness, and increasing skeletal muscle readiness[1].

Norepinephrine is released during a stressful event by activation of the brain stem.

Low norepinephrine is associated with attention-deficit/hyperactivity disorder and depression.1,5

Tyrosine is the precursor to norepinephrine (noradrenaline), epinephrine (adrenaline), and thyroid hormones. Tyrosine can be synthesized in the body from phenylalanine, except in premature infants and in Phenylketonuria. Common food sources for phenylalanine include: pork liver, soybeans, soy products, dry skim milk, dairy, fish, meat, poultry, almonds, peanuts, brazil nuts, pecans, pumpkin seeds, sesame seeds, lima beans, chickpeas, and lentils4. Common food sources of tyrosine include: Meat, dairy, eggs, almonds, avocados, bananas, fish, wheat, oats, lima beans, pumpkin seeds, and sesame seeds4.

In the study by Van Winkle, et al they found that endogenous toxic metabolites interfered with neurotransmission, causing periodic depression, and overexcited synapses with excess norepinephrine causing mild anxiety to violent behavior. After the norepinephrine has been depleted, depression returned. There is a definite connection between emotions and neurotransmission. The dynamics of neurotransmitter levels in the brain need to be analyzed with respect to time. During periods of excess levels of norepinephrine in the brain, there are elevations in mood. After the norepinephrine reserves have been depleted, depression follows.

"The continual suppression of emotions during fight or flight reactions results in atrophy and endogenous toxicosis in noradrenergic neurons. Toxic metabolites interfere with neurotransmission, causing depression. During periodic detoxification crises, excess norepinephrine floods synapses, overexcite postsynaptic neurons, and cause symptoms ranging from mild anxiety to violent behavior. When toxic metabolites, which may include excess dopamine, epinephrine, serotonin, gamma-aminobutyric acid, peptides, amino acids, and various metabolic waste products, are bound to noradrenergic receptor sites, these sites become unavailable to norepinephrine. Excitation of postsynaptic neurons is diminished and depression returns16."

The dynamics of neurotransmitter levels must be analyzed with respect to time. Changes in neurotransmitter levels begin with an initial reaction followed by a loss of neurotransmitter reserves if they cannot be replaced at least at the same rate by which they are depleted.

Balancing the level of norepinephrine is tricky because an increase in norepinephrine levels can lead to an increase in epinephrine levels if norepinephrine methylase is being constantly activated by a demand for epinephrine during anxiety and the fight or flight response. Norepinephrine has a stimulating effect on the stimulatory adrenergic receptors. Epinephrine is 5-10 times more stimulating to the adrenergic receptors than norepinephrine. A low level can cause depression and migraine headaches. A higher than normal level can cause insomnia, anxiety, etc. A very high level can cause increased aggression and perhaps violence. This statement appears to be in conflict with the study13, in which norepinephrine levels were found to be low. This can be explained as follows. The fight or flight response calls for an increase in epinephrine. Epinephrine is metabolized from norepinephrine so that norepinephrine needs to be produced first in order to produce epinephrine. Therefore, the demand for epinephrine will initially increase the levels of norepinephrine, followed by a decrease in norepinephrine when it is metabolized to epinephrine.

Chemical stimulants such as caffeine, ephedrine, pseudoephedrine, etc., can produce the fight or flight response, which can result in mania, exaggerated aggression, and perhaps violence if serotonin in the brain is low.

Mania and aggression occurs when the serotonin levels in the brain are low and the norepinephrine levels in the brain are high15. It appears that one of the best solutions to excessive norepinephrine and epinephrine production may be to decrease the anxiety and fight or flight response through psychotherapy, meditation, yoga, and other stress reducing modalities. If these methods are not effective or not used, maintaining an adequately high level of serotonin through diet and supplementation is vitally important.

For individuals who are chronically depressed and in attention-deficit/hyperactivity disorder, the administration of tyrosine or phenylalanine may be required. This should be done carefully and with attention to the neurotransmitter dynamics within time, to avoid promoting an increase of epinephrine.

Tyramine causes norepinephrine to be released from sympathetic nerve ending and epinephrine from the adrenal glands. Initially, this release results in increased sympathetic stimulation, which causes higher blood pressure, insomnia, increased aggression in some cases, increased glucose release, increased metabolism, inhibition of the G.I. tract, and increased cardiovascular activity. Increased sympathetic stimulation can also result in a depletion of serotonin. The final result is a depletion of norepinephrine, epinephrine, and serotonin reserves. An individual's activity, as a result of tyramine intake, may initially go from mania to depression and migraine headaches later on.

Cheese contains high amounts of tyrosine and tyramine. The high amount of tyrosine allows the norepinephrine and epinephrine levels to elevate in those who are suffering from anxiety and leading stressful and active lifestyles. The high amount of tyramine, which will be discussed in greater detail later, causes the serotonin levels to decrease. The result is mania, exaggerated aggression, and often violence. Cheddar cheese contains 42.5 mg of tyramine per ounce of cheese. An amount of 10-25 mg of tyramine can cause a severe reaction. Regardless of media advertising, cheese is not natural. It does not exist in nature. It is man-made.

Tyramine is a vaso-active amino acid that displaces norepinephrine from the nerve endings and epinephrine from the adrenal glands. Monoamine oxidase is in the gastrointestinal tract and inactivates tyramine. There is an adverse reaction when there is either too much tyramine or too little monoamine oxidase. The tyramine content in foods vary greatly due to different processing, aging, fermentation, ripening and/or contamination. Many foods that contain small amounts of tyramine develop large amounts of tyramine if the food products were left to spoil, age (not fresh), or fermented. The emphasis is placed on FRESH FOODS. Fruits that are permissible should be very fresh. Avoid leftovers kept in the refrigerator especially meats, dry packages mixes and can products (prepared foods), yeast extracts, and protein extracts. Remember, foods increase in their tyramine content as they age or ferment. For example, bananas are permissible if they are fresh, not if they are overripe.

Tyramine can also be produced by bacteria in the gastrointestinal track. Helicobactor pylori can produce large amounts of tyramine in the gut. Various bacteria in the gut can cause an increase in the production of tyramine.

The brain converts tryptophan to serotonin. Serotonin itself cannot transport into the brain, it needs to be manufactured there. Tryptophan requires an albumin carrier to transport into the brain. Tryptophan competes with amino acids and fatty acids to attach to the albumin carrier. High carbohydrates will increase the body's ability to transport tryptophan into the brain. So, when the brain is low in serotonin, it creates an appetite for carbohydrates.

Mild tyramine reactions can occur with approximately 6 mg of tyramine. Severe reactions can occur with 10-25 mg tyramine of tyramine.

Approximate tyramine contents of food:

Cheddar cheese = 1.5 mg/g (42.5 mg/ounce)

Blue Stilton = 0.2 mg/g (5.6 mg/ounce)

Gouda = 0.02 mg/g (0.56 mg/ounce)

Beer = 0.02 mg/g (0.56 mg/ounce)

Wine = 0.025 mg/g (0.71 mg/ounce)

Yeast Extracts = 2 mg/g (56.6 mg/ounce)

Food to Avoid:
Any Food that is aged, cultured, or fermented
Cheeses
Chocolate
Eggs, If allergic
Raw Onions & Garlic
Cooked Onions & Garlic (small quantities only)
Citrus and Citric Acid
Mustard
Red wine
Berries (most kinds with thick skin)
Over-ripened fruits
Avocado
Monosodium Glutamate (MSG)
Nitrates & Nitrites
Meat tenderizers
Salad bars that spray with sulfites
Aspartame (nutrasweet)
Saccharin (includes toothpaste and mouthwash)
Smoked/cured meats
Cold cuts containing nitrates, etc.
Frankfurters containing nitrates, etc.
Food preservatives
Some drugs can trigger a migraine, Depression, etc. depending upon your sensitivity to those drugs
Nuts and nut butters in large quantity
Beans in large quantity
Tomatoes in large quantity
Yeast and brewers extracts
Sourdough
Kelp, Seaweed, Shell fish, and other Fish containing significant amounts of lithium
Alcoholic beverages including beer
Excessive use of coffee or tea containing caffeine

Tempeh, Tomari, Yogurt, Umbusi, Soy sauce, Miso, Vinegar (fermented)

Tobacco

Frequent use of amphetamines

Frequent use of barbituates

Frequent use 1of recreation drugs

Decaffeinated coffee (only 50% less caffeine)

Excessive exposure to fluorescent lighting

Aged, marinated, or pickled meats

Non-fresh meats or fish

Protein extracts

Tofu

Wheat if there is intestinal Candida overgrowth or allergy

Paint fumes & other chemical fumes

Food to Eat:

The following food are relatively safe to eat unless your are allergic to any of them.

Bell & Evans Frozen Fully Cooked Grilled Chicken Breasts, Frozen, Ingredients: boneless, skinless,chicken beasts, water, sea salt, rice starch.

Lundberg Organic brown rice, short or long grain, Ingredients: organic short or long grain brown rice.

Lundberg Organic brown basmati rice, Ingredients: organic California brown basmati rice.

Minute Ready to Serve brown rice, Ingredients: water, whole grain brown rice, soybean oil, salt, soy lecithin.

Shiloh Farms Organic Potato Fakes, instant, Ingredients: organic potato flakes, monoglycerides, and diglycerides (from organic palm oil).

Any brand, Instant Oatmeal, Ingredients: whole grain instant oats.

Envirokids Corn Puffs Gorilla Munch, Ingredients: corn meal, evaporated cane juice, sea salt.

Nature's Path Organic Crispy Rice, Ingredients: brown rice flour, evaporated cane juice, sea salt, molasses.

Back to Nature Classic Granola, Ingredients: whole grain rolled oats, evaporated cane juice, pineapple juice, peach juice, pear juice concentrate, vitamin E, natural flavor.

Quaker Rice Cakes, Ingredients: whole grain brown rice.

So Delicious Unsweetened Coconut Milk, Ingredients: organic coconut milk, (water, organic coconut cream), calcium phosphate, magnesium phosphate, carrageenan, guar gum, vitamin A palmitate, vitamin D, selenium, zinc oxide, folic acid, vitamin B12.

Spinach, Arugala, Romain Lettuce, broccoli, zucchini, corn, carrots, and many other vegetables, except raw garlic, onions, and radishes.

Cold Pressed Olive Oil.

Coffee, unflavored, organic.

Organic Fat-Free Milk if not allergic.

Organic Butter in small quantities.

Ice Cream, vanilla.

Spices: parsley, oregano, basil, pepper, salt, in small quantity.

Sweetener: sugar in small quantity.

The following should also be avoided:
Excessive exposure to fluorescent lighting
Paint fumes & other chemical fumes

Individuals suffering from anxiety and a stressful lifestyle should follow a low tyrosine diet. Tyrosine containing foods should be divided into portions throughout the day. They should also look into stress reduction techniques such as psychotherapy, special relaxation tapes and techniques, exercise, meditation, YOGA, deep breathing, biofeedback, etc.

Exercise

Introduction

Daily exercise is an important part of this program. Exercise sets your metabolic rate, increases your blood flow, reduces your stress, and plays an important role in oxygenating your cells. Check with your family physician first. Choose the type(s) of exercise you enjoy. Walking (briskly) everyday for 20 minutes should constitute an adequate amount of exercise.

Aerobic exercise continuously uses large muscle groups. It also elevates the heart rate and breathing for a sustained period of time. Examples include walking, jogging/running, swimming, rowing, stair climbing, bicycling, cross-country skiing, step and dance exercise classes, roller and ice skating, tennis, racquetball, and squash. You should cross train (alternating between types of exercises) to reduce the possibility of repetition injuries.

A weak heart cannot pump as much blood as a healthy heart when the muscle contracts. A weak heart will compensate by pumping more blood each minute, causing the heart to age and weaken prematurely. A healthy or well-conditioned heart may have a heart rate of 50 beats, which pumps the same amount of blood per minute as a weaker heart pumps in 80 beats. The difference is 30 beats per minute, 1,800 beats per hour, 43,200 beats per day, and 15,778,800 beats per year.

Any form of exercise, which requires you to use your muscles will cause your body to burn fat. The best exercises for burning fat are those which can be done continuously and involve most of the muscle groups (especially the large muscles of the hips and legs). The more muscles you use, and the longer the time you use them, the more fat you will burn.

Exercise actually regulates your appetite helping you eat fewer calories and it increases metabolism. Moderate exercise increases your metabolic rate (calorie burning) by a factor of 8 for several hours after the exercise. The movement involved with exercise requires you to use your muscles, which causes the muscle to maintain or increase in size and strength. Every pound of muscle requires 50-100 calories per day to sustain itself. Fat is burned almost exclusively in your muscles. Therefore, maintaining your muscle is important to losing body fat. Without exercise, you will lose muscle and reduce your ability to burn fat. Muscles have very specific enzymes, which burn fat. People who exercise regularly have far more fat-burning enzymes in their muscles than people who don't exercise.

Exercise affects various hormone levels, which are related to fat storage such as insulin, adrenaline, and cortisol. Endorphins, (morphine-like chemicals), are secreted with exercise, which help reduce fat storage and alleviate stress. Exercise also increases food transit time through the intestines, which reduces the chances for digestive disorders and bowel cancer. Exercise also improves your sleeping patterns, energy level, and overall feeling of well-being.

During aerobic exercise, your body uses fat and carbohydrates/sugar for energy. A long duration of low to moderate intensity exercise is the best way to lose fat. Higher intensity exercises burn more carbohydrates/sugars than fat. When you exercise at 60% of your maximum heart rate, approximately 50% of the calories you burn come from fat. When you exercise at 80% of your maximum heart rate, only 40% of calories you burn come from fat.

Aerobic exercise does not provide much muscle toning/firming. Resistance exercise (weight training) provides muscle toning/firming. Aerobic exercise does not require a high degree of concentration. So, you may want to read, listen to music or educational tapes, or watch TV.

Consult your doctor before starting any exercise program, especially if you have a history of health problems, haven't had a recent physical checkup, or are pregnant or lactating.

Duration

Ten to 60 minutes of exercise will provide great benefits. If you want to lose body fat, the longer the duration of exercise, the better. You should exercise at least 30 to 60 minutes. Your fitness level can improve with an exercise duration of 10 minutes, provided you repeat the exercise 2 to 3 times a day, 5 days a week.

For general fitness, 30 minutes of exercise is adequate, repeated 3 times or more per week.

Warming up before your exercise is important to prevent injuries. The warm up increases blood flow and oxygen throughout the body and raises body temperature. You can warm up by stretching, light calisthenics, or pedaling at very low speed. You should warm up for 2 to 5 minutes.

Cooling down is also important to prevent injuries. Stopping suddenly after an intense exercise can cause an accumulation of blood in the extremities, which causes the heart to exert more force and increases the probability of soreness in the muscles. To cool down, gradually, reduce your exercise for 2 to 5 minutes.

Intensity

Your heart rate is the most accurate method of measuring the intensity of your exercise. You can determine your heart rate by taking your pulse for 15 seconds and multiplying it by 4. Heart rate monitors are easier to continuously monitor your heart rate. You can also judge the intensity of your exercise by the 'talk test.' You should be able to talk comfortably while you are exercising. If you are recovering from an illness or injury, or are significantly overweight, you should begin with a low to moderate intensity exercise of 60% of your maximum heat rate.

Maximum heart rate (MHR) = 220 - Age.

Multiply MHR times 0.60 for 60%, etc.

60% to 70% of MHR = Weight Management Zone.

70% to 80% of MHR = Aerobic Zone.

80% to 90% of MHR = Aerobic Threshold Zone.

Moderately intense activities include: brisk walking (3-4 mph), cycling (10 mph), swimming or calisthenics, racket sports or table tennis, golf (without cart), housecleaning*, raking leaves*, dancing*, playing actively with children*.

*Considered moderate only if they are performed at an intensity comparable to brisk walking. (Journal of the American Medical Association 273:402:1995.)

Frequency

You should exercise 3 to 7 days per week. If your goal is to maintain fitness, 3 to 5 days per week will be adequate. If your goal is fat loss, then 6 to 7 low impact workouts per week should be adequate. The more often you perform aerobic exercise the more important it is to cross train. It is important to gradually increase your duration, intensity, and frequency, especially if you are under-conditioned, overweight, elderly, or rehabilitating from an injury or illness. If in doubt, go easier, shorter, and slower.

You should keep a record of your workouts and body fat percentage measurements to see how far you have progressed.

Body Fat

You cannot determine good health by measuring weight alone because it does not differentiate between body fat and lean body mass (muscle). Too much fat is called obesity, and puts a person at risk for many serious medical conditions including heart disease, diabetes and cancer. Obesity means an excess of body fat regardless of weight.

According to the National Institute of Health, 1999, the healthy range for women 20-39 years of age is 20.5% to 35.0%. For women 40-59 years of age the range is 21.3% to 35.8%. For female seniors 60-79 years of age the range is 22.1% to 36.6%. The Institute warns that there are specific health risks associated with low body fat percents, especially for women and children. This is primarily due to endocrine function (hormone production). For men 20-39 years of age the range is 8.9% to 21.2%. For men 40-59 years of age, the range is 10.2% to 22.9%. For male seniors 60-79 years of age the range is 11.9%-24.5%.

Weight Management

Your primary goal should be to maintain your weight. Your secondary goal may be to lose weight. It is important to make your goals a long-term part of your lifestyle.

There are no quick fixes in weight loss. Biologically, humans have a predisposition for building up fat deposits for survival in times of famine, especially females. A woman's body is designed to protect her and her potential fetus. Women have more enzymes for storing fat and fewer enzymes for burning fat. The hormone Estrogen promotes fat storing enzymes. Frequent dieting slows down your metabolic rate, reduces your lean muscular tissue, and increases body fat.

The Basal Metabolic Rate (BMR) is the daily caloric requirement needed to maintain lean mass. If you decrease your caloric intake below your BMR, the body thinks it is in a state of starvation and begins to rid itself of whatever material that consumes the most calories, which is your lean muscle tissue. Calories are burned in your muscle. So, decreasing your muscle mass will decrease your ability to burn calories. This is why dieting alone will cause you to decrease your lean muscle tissue and increase body fat.

Before the 1950's the average American woman consumed 3,000 to 5,000 calories per day. Today the average American woman consumes less than 1,500 calories per day and is on some type of weight loss program. In the 1970's one fourth of the population of the United States was considered obese. Today one third of the population is considered obese. We have become a society more and more dependent upon weight-loss diets, appetite suppressants, and commercial weight loss centers. As a result, we have become a more unhealthy society.

To lose weight, or more properly to lose body fat, you must enter into a program of aerobic (fat burning) exercise and good nutrition.

Perspiration

The skin is a vitally important organ that eliminates toxins through perspiration. Exercises that cause perspiration will facilitate the elimination of toxins.

Desktop Yoga

A modern style for those who have little time and for those who have little energy

One of the primary purposes of yoga and meditation is to "still" the mind. This was difficult even for the sages that developed yoga. Today's society is many times more stressful than our grandparents. With radio, television, computers, e-mail, cell phones, and other technologies, minds are constantly being stressed. When traditional yoga is performed in a stressful society, the stressful mind may continue to "chatter," even within the postures. Furthermore, most people don't have the time to practice yoga.

The Desktop Yoga style was developed by Dr. John A. Allocca in response to the growing need for a yoga style that can be performed successfully in a stressful society. It brings the scattered, stressful, chattering, mind into focus by integrating coordinated breathing and slow movements within each posture. The mind must focus its attention on coordinating the breathing and slow movements, which removes it's attention from the "chatter." The result is a yoga practice that "stills" the mind and creates relaxation. The bilateral movements are also designed to stimulate the release of stored emotional traumas from the limbic system in the brain, creating a greater sense of peace and well-being. The slow movements thin the fluid in the joints and allow even better stretching than postures without movements. Desktop yoga can be performed while sitting in an armless chair. It is a low-intensity, short-duration series of postures for those who have little time and for those who have little energy. The routine will take approximately 15 minutes to perform, not including the meditation.

Breathing

Sit straight facing forward with your feet together.

Slowly and deeply inhale from your abdomen first, then your chest.

Slowly exhale completely and push from your abdomen.

During Asanas (postures), you can keep your eyes closed or open. I prefer closed. I prefer to take 3 slow, deep breaths for each posture.

Three breaths will take about 15 seconds. As you advance, your breaths can be longer.

Relaxing Into a Posture

Don't push your muscles into a stretch. Allow them to stretch by relaxing your muscles. Don't stretch to the point of pain. If you experience pain, release a little or come out of the posture.

Counting Your Breaths

I count my breaths by saying (mentally) "Om" during the inhalation and the number during the exhalation. For example, Om (inhale), one (exhale), Om (inhale), two (exhale), Om (inhale), three (exhale). If you are in a group, just say (mentally) Om (inhale), then (exhale) and allow the instructor to tell you when to release.

Movement Cycles

All movements should be done slowly while concentrating on your breaths. Do not move quickly. This is not an aerobic exercise. If, for example, you are rotating your head from center to the left, you should inhale as you are rotating your head. The inhalation should take the entire time that you are slowly rotating.

Warm-up Exercises

Rubbing Hands

Rub hands together vigorously.

Neck Roll

Roll neck clockwise one complete rotation. Roll neck counter clockwise one complete rotation. Repeat 3 times.

Small Arm Circles

Hands and arms out to the side. Make small circular rotations with hands 3 times. Reverse direction and repeat 3 times.

Shoulder Roll

Roll shoulders forward 3 times.
Roll shoulders backward 3 times.
Lift shoulders up and down 3 times.

Waist Twisting

Arms horizontal and to the front at shoulder level. Rotate from side to side, keeping head and hips forward 3 times.

Arms Up and Down

Inhale, arms to the front and up to the sky. Exhale arms down to the side. Repeat 3 times.

Horizontal Adduction Arm Cross

Arms out to the sides. Then move to the front and back, alternating which hand is on top each time. Repeat 3 times.

Desktop Yoga Postures (Asanas)

Neck Rotation Posture

Sit straight facing forward with your feet together.

Inhale deeply.

a. Exhale as you slowly rotate your head to the left while pushing your chin gently with your right hand.

b. Inhale as you slowly rotate your head to the center.

Repeat movement cycles a and b 3 times.

Inhale deeply.

a. Exhale as you slowly rotate your head to the right while pushing your chin gently with your left hand.

b. Inhale as you slowly rotate your head to the center.

Repeat movement cycles a and b 3 times.

Relax and breathe into the posture.

Concentrate on your breathing.

Neck Stretch Posture

Sit straight facing forward with your feet together.

Inhale deeply.

Bring your left hand up and around to the right side of your head.

Inhale deeply.

a. Exhale as you slowly pull your head to the left with your left hand.

b. Inhale as you slowly bring your head to the center.

Repeat movement cycles a and b 3 times.

Inhale deeply.

a. Exhale as you slowly pull your head to the right with your right hand.

b. Inhale as you slowly bring your head to the center.
Repeat movement cycles a and b 3 times.
Relax and breathe into the posture.
Concentrate on your breathing.

Seated Posture with Arms Stretched Up

Sit straight facing forward with your feet together.

Extend your arms along the sides of your body with palms facing your thighs and fingers pointing down.

a. Inhale as you raise your arms to the sky with palms facing forward.

b. Exhale as you allow your shoulders to lower slightly, while keeping your arms vertical.

Repeat movement cycles a and b 3 times.

Relax and breathe into the posture.

Concentrate on your breathing.

Seated Posture with Bound Hands

Sit straight facing forward with your feet together.

Raise your arms just above your head, interlock your fingers and rotate your palms facing up.

a. Inhale as you push your hands and arms up to the sky.

b. Exhale as your allow your hands and arms to lower slightly, while keeping your arms vertical.

Repeat movement cycles a and b 3 times.

Relax and breathe into the posture.

Concentrate on your breathing.

Elevated Arm Stretch Posture

Sit straight facing forward with your feet together.

Bring your left arm straight up.

Bend your elbow and allow your left hand to come down behind your head.

Hold your left elbow with your right hand and pull slightly.

a. Inhale as you slowly lean slightly backward.

b. Exhale as you slowly lean forward.

Repeat movement cycles a and b 3 times.

Relax and breathe into the posture.

Concentrate on your breathing.

Repeat for the other side.

Posterior Hand Clasp Posture

Sit straight facing forward with your feet together.

Clasp your hands behind your back.

a. Inhale as you lift your chest.

b. Exhale as you drop your shoulders and hands.

Repeat movement cycles a and b 3 to 7 times.

Relax and breathe into the posture.

Concentrate on your breathing.

Horizontal Adduction Posture

(Adduction is towards the body, Abduction is away from the body)

Sit straight facing forward with your feet together.

Bring your left arm across your chest parallel to the floor with your palms facing downward.

Bring your right hand to your left arm between your shoulder and elbow.

a. Inhale as your pull slightly.

b. Exhale as you slowly release your arm slightly.

Repeat movement cycles a and b 3 times.

Relax and breathe into the posture.

Concentrate on your breathing.

Repeat for the other side.

Seated Cobra Posture

Sit straight facing forward with your feet together.

Place your palms on the seat.

a. Inhale as you sweep up, arch your back, and tilt your head back if possible.

b. Exhale as you lower your head down and arch your back down.

Repeat movement cycles a and b 3 times.

Relax and breathe into the posture.

Concentrate on your breathing.

Seated Back Bend Posture

Sit straight facing forward with your feet together and your hand on your hips.

Inhale as you lift your chest and shoulders.

Exhale as you lean back as far as you can go without pain or falling back with your head gently tilted back.

Inhale deeply.

a. Exhale as you slowly swing your torso in an arc to the left.

b. Inhale as you slowly swing your torso in an arc to the center.

c. Exhale as you slowly swing your torso in an arc to the right.

Repeat movement cycles a, b, and c, 3 times - always returning to center before moving left or right.

Relax and breathe into the posture.

Concentrate on your breathing.

Seated Leg Elevation Posture

Sit straight facing forward with your feet together.

Place your arms to the side with your palms resting on the seat.

a. Inhale as you slowly raise your legs.

b. Exhale as you slowly lower your legs.

Repeat movement cycles a and b 3 times.

Relax and breathe into the posture.

Concentrate on your breathing.

Seated Spinal Twist Posture

Sit straight facing forward with feet together.

Rotate your torso to the left.

Place your left palm on the seat behind you.

Bring your right hand over your left leg and rest your palm on the seat behind you with your head up.

a. Inhale as you slowly rotate your torso to the left.

b. Exhale as you slowly rotate your torso to the center.

Repeat movement cycles a and b 3 times.

Relax and breathe into the posture.

Concentrate on your breathing.

Repeat for the other side.

Seated Forward Fold Posture

Sit straight facing forward with your feet together.

a. Inhale as you raise your arms straight up to the sky with palms facing forward.

b. Exhale as you slowly bend forward with your arms down and forward as far as possible while keeping your head down.

Repeat movement cycles a and b 3 times.

Relax and breathe into the posture.

Concentrate on your breathing.

Seated Leg Stretch Posture

Sit straight facing forward with your feet together.

Grasp your right ankle and bend your knee.

a. Inhale and bring your ankle as far back as possible.

b. Exhale and release slightly.

Repeat movement cycles a and b 3 times.

Relax and breathe into the posture.

Concentrate on your breathing.

Seated Half Lotus Posture

Sit straight facing forward with your feet together.

Bend your left leg and place your left foot over your right thigh.

a. Inhale as you raise your knee up.

b. Exhale as you allow your knee to push down while keeping your head up.

Repeat movement cycles a and b 3 times.

Relax and breathe into the posture.

Concentrate on your breathing.

Repeat for the other side.

Pranic Breathing Meditation

Sit straight facing forward with your feet apart.

Begin meditating by closing your eyes and imagining someone who will help you to feel love. Open your heart and feel love, unconditional love for people, animals, plants, and all of God's creations. Feeling love is the most important part of this meditation.

Imagine that there is a hollow tube about 1-1/2 inches in diameter that extends from the top of your head, through your body along your spine to the bottom of your spine.

Inhale slowly and deeply. Expand your diaphragm and belly first, then allow your chest to expand as you draw in prana through the top and bottom of the hollow tube.

The inhalation should take about 7 seconds.

Exhale slowly and deeply by contracting your diaphragm and belly first, then allowing your chest to contract as you concentrate the prana in your hara.

The exhalation should take about 7 seconds.

Repeat the inhalations and exhalations deeply for 7 breaths. After the 7 deep breathes, begin to breathe normally and regularly.

Concentrate on the regularity of your breathing and the flow of prana through the tube from both directions and the concentration of prana in your hara. It is not unusual to feel palpitation in your heart as the energy flows through your body. This is the life-giving energy that cleanses and rebuilds your mind and body.

As thoughts or pictures come into your mind, allow them to be the focus of your attention. Allow them to enter and exit your consciousness freely.

In meditation, you will meet and melt away emotional and mental blocks, as well as physical tensions. You will generally feel peaceful and refreshed after meditating.

It is beneficial to meditate at least a few times per week. The actual time of each meditation will vary - don't be concerned with time.

In this altered state of consciousness you will be able to be in contact with nature, and the universe around you. The possibilities of what you can do in this state are limitless.

Healthy Gourmet Wheat, Gluten, Dairy, Egg, and Yeast, Free Recipes

Breakfast

Almond Breakfast Cereal or Snack

1/4 cup almond flour

1/4 cup cashew nuts, chopped coarsely

1/4 teaspoon ground cinnamon

Dash of nutmeg

1/8 cup water

Cashew Breakfast Cereal or Snack

1/4 cup almond flour

1/4 cup cashew nuts, chopped coarsely

1/4 teaspoon ground cinnamon

Dash of nutmeg

1/8 cup water

Appetizers

Baba Ghannouj

2 large eggplants (about 2 pounds)

1/4 cup lemon juice (not for migraineur's)

3 tablespoons cold pressed sesame oil

2 cloves garlic, finely mashed

4 tablespoons sesame seeds

1/2 teaspoon sea salt

1/2 teaspoon black pepper

Preheat oven to 450O F.

Peel and grate the eggplants. Bake grated eggplant in a casserole with cover for 45 minutes. Remove from oven and let stand until cool. Simmer garlic in oil a few minutes or until lightly brown. Mix all ingredients with an electric mixer for 1 minute. Place mixture in a bowl, cover and refrigerate for one day. Remove from refrigerator 30 minutes before serving. Serve with vegetables you like except potatoes or carrots

Bean Dip

3 tablespoons cold pressed olive oil

2 cloves garlic, chopped

30 oz. refried beans

3/4 cup water

1/2 teaspoon basil

1/4 teaspoon black pepper

1/2 teaspoon oregano

1/2 teaspoon parsley

1/2 teaspoon sea salt

Using a deep skillet, sauté the garlic in olive oil until dark brown. Lower heat and add remaining ingredients. Cook for another 5 minutes. Serve with vegetables you like except potatoes or carrots

Bean Salad

16 oz. kidney beans, drained

16 oz. garbanzo beans, drained

2 cloves garlic, finely chopped

1/2 cup oil and lemon dressing recipe (not for migraineur's)

Mix the above ingredients together and serve.

Hummus

16 oz. garbanzo beans

3 tablespoons cold pressed olive oil

1 clove garlic or more, finely mashed

1 teaspoon parsley

3 tablespoons lemon juice (not for migraineur's)

dash of cayenne pepper

1/4 cup water

      Add garbanzo beans, sesame oil, garlic, lemon juice, cayenne, and 1/4 cup of water to a food processor. Process until smooth. Add more water if mixture is too thick. Allow to chill in the refrigerator for at least one hour. Spread on a flat platter and garnish with parley. Serve with vegetables you like except potatoes or carrots.

Indian Red Relish

2 cloves garlic, chopped

1 onion, chopped (optional)

8 oz. tomato puree

3 tablespoons cold pressed olive oil

1/2 teaspoon cayenne pepper or less

1 teaspoon turmeric

1/2 teaspoon coriander

1/2 teaspoon cumin

1/4 teaspoon salt

1/4 teaspoon black pepper

1 tablespoon lemon juice (not for migraineur's)

1/4 cup water

      Mix all above ingredients. Serve with vegetables you like except potatoes or carrots.

Salmon Spread

1/2 pound salmon, cooked

3 teaspoons cold pressed olive oil

1/8 teaspoon cayenne pepper

1/2 teaspoon basil

1/4 cup lemon juice (not for migraineur's)

1/4 teaspoon sea salt

1/8 teaspoon black pepper

      Blend salmon in food processor. Gradually add oil. Add the remaining ingredients and continue blending until mixture is smooth. Cover and store in refrigerator. Serve chilled.

Soups

Bean and Mushroom Soup

4 tablespoons cold pressed olive oil

2 large cloves garlic, chopped

1/2 tablespoon organic butter

1 bunch scallions, chopped

3/4 pound mushrooms, sliced

4 cups water

1/2 teaspoon sea salt

1/2 teaspoon black pepper

Dash of cayenne pepper

1 tablespoon parsley

1 tablespoon basil

1 tablespoon oregano

2 cans white beans, drained and washed

In a 6-quart pot, sauté the garlic, olive oil, and butter at medium heat until the garlic is lightly brown. Add the scallions and continue to cook for another minute. Add the mushrooms and continue cooking for another 5 minutes. Add the remaining ingredients and simmer for 20 minutes. Remove the pot from the stove and puree the soup with a hand blender. Caution soup is hot. Be very careful while pureeing. Serve hot.

Vegetable Soup

8 cups water (3 quarts)

1 cup brown or green lentils

1 pound mushrooms, sliced

4 stalks celery, sliced

2 cloves garlic, chopped

2 tablespoons parsley

2 teaspoon basil

1/8 teaspoon or more cayenne pepper

1/2 teaspoon black pepper

1 teaspoon sea salt

Bring water to a boil in an 8-quart pot. Add ingredients and allow to a boil for 3 minutes. Lower heat and simmer for 1 hour. Stir occasionally. Serve hot. Leftover soup can be frozen. Serves 6 to 8 people.

Spaghetti Squash Soup

3 tablespoons cold pressed olive oil

2 cloves garlic, chopped

1 spaghetti squash

Chinese cabbage or bok choy (optional)

1 red bell pepper, chopped

1 green bell pepper, chopped

1 onion, chopped (optional)

1/2 pound mushroom, sliced

1 teaspoon sea salt

1/2 teaspoon black pepper

1 teaspoon parsley

1 teaspoon basil

1/2 teaspoon oregano

1/8 teaspoon or more cayenne pepper

Water

Bake the spaghetti squash in an over for 1 hour at 375 degrees F. Remove it from the oven and allow it to cool. Cut the squash in half lengthwise. Remove the seeds. With a fork, strip the strands of squash from the shell.

Sauté garlic in olive oil until lightly brown in an 8-quart pot at medium heat. Add onions, peppers and mushrooms. Continue cooking for about 5 minutes. Add the remaining ingredients. Add water to about 1 inch above the ingredients. Cook for 1 hour at low heat.

Snacks

Zucchini

1 raw zucchini
Cold pressed olive oil
Sea salt
Black pepper
Oregano

Skin the zucchini. Cut it into slices that are about 1/4 inch thick. Lay them out on a plate. Add a few drops of olive oil and other ingredients on top of each. Serve cold.

Mushrooms

Raw button mushrooms
Cold pressed olive oil
Sea salt
Black pepper
Oregano

Cut in half. Lay them out on a plate with the cut side up. Add a few drops of olive oil and other ingredients on top of each. Serve cold.

Vegetables

Any raw vegetables you like except potatoes or carrots
Cold pressed olive oil
Sea salt
Black pepper
Oregano

Cut the vegetables as desired. Lay them out on a plate. Add a few drops of olive oil and other ingredients on top of each. Serve cold.

Sauces

Curry Sauce

3 tablespoons cold pressed olive oil

2 cloves garlic, chopped

16 oz. tomato puree

1/2 teaspoon black pepper

1/2 teaspoon cardamom

A dash or more of cayenne

1 teaspoon turmeric

1/2 teaspoon coriander

1/2 teaspoon cumin

1/4 teaspoon sea salt

Sauté garlic and oil in a 3-quart pot. Add remaining ingredients. Simmer for 10 to 20 minutes.

Marinara Sauce

3 tablespoons cold pressed olive oil

4 large cloves garlic, chopped

1 onion, chopped (optional)

28 oz. whole tomatoes

6 fresh basil leaves, chopped

1 tablespoon oregano

1 tablespoon parsley

1 tablespoon basil

1/2 teaspoon sea salt

1/2 teaspoon black pepper

Dash of cayenne pepper

The origins of marinara sauce, is that the sauce was made in Naples for the sailors when they returned from the sea. The sauce does not contain fish or anything from the sea.

In an 6-quart pot, sauté' garlic and olive oil at medium heat until the garlic is soft and lightly browned. Crush the tomatoes with a fork or puree the tomatoes in a blender. Add remaining ingredients except the basil. Bring to a boil, then lower heat to a simmer and cook until thickened approximately 20 to 30 minutes. Add basil just before serving. Serve over vegetables. Serves 2-4 people.

Garlic and Oil Sauce

3 tablespoons cold pressed olive oil

2 cloves garlic, finely chopped

1 teaspoon parsley

1/2 teaspoon oregano

1/2 teaspoon sea salt

1/8 teaspoon black pepper

1/4 cup soup broth

Sauté garlic until brown; let cool for 2 minutes. Add rest of ingredients and continue cooking for 5-10 minutes. Add vegetables.

Pesto Sauce

2 cups fresh basil leaves

1 cup parsley

1/4 cup cold pressed olive oil

2 cloves garlic, pressed

Mix in a food processor or blender, heat mildly and pour over 1/2 to 1 pound of brown rice or quinoa pasta. Serves 2 people.

Tahini Sauce & Dressing

1 cup sesame tahini

1/2 cup or more water

4 tablespoons lemon juice (not for migraineur's)

4 tablespoons cold pressed olive oil

1/2 teaspoon sea salt

1/2 teaspoon black pepper

Mix above ingredients in a blender until smooth. If used as a salad dressing, add more water.

Tomato Sauce

4 tablespoons cold pressed olive oil

2 cloves garlic, chopped

2 onions, chopped (optional)

32 oz. tomato puree

1/2 pound mushrooms, sliced

1 tablespoon oregano

1 tablespoon fresh basil

1 tablespoon parsley

1/2 tablespoon sea salt

1/2 teaspoon black pepper

1/2 teaspoon or less cayenne pepper

6 fresh basil leaves, chopped

1 pound any vegetables you like except potatoes or carrots

In an 8-quart pot sauté garlic in oil until brown. Add remaining ingredients. Simmer 2 hours, stirring every 15 minutes. Serves over vegetables.

Main Dishes

Baked Tilapia

Fresh tilapia

Cold pressed olive oil

Sea salt

Black pepper

Garlic powder

Oregano

Preheat oven to 350 degrees F.

Add a little olive oil to the bottom of a 24-ounce au gratin baking dish or a Pyrex 9.5 x 15.2 x 2.2 inch baking dish. Place the tilapia (3 tilapia in the Pyrex dish) with the side with the red marks, down into the baking dish. Sprinkle some olive oil over the tilapia. Sprinkle some salt, pepper, garlic powder and oregano over the top of the tilapia. Cover with aluminum foil. Bake in the oven at 350 degrees F for 30 minutes. Each tilapia feeds one.

Chicken Creole

3 tablespoons cold pressed olive oil

3 cloves garlic, chopped

2 cloves of garlic, chopped

1 green pepper, chopped

2 pounds chicken breasts, cut into 3/4" pieces

2 stalks of celery, diced

1 large bay leaf

1 teaspoon basil

1/8 teaspoon black pepper

1/8 teaspoon cayenne pepper

1 teaspoon parsley

1/2 teaspoon sea salt

16 oz. tomato puree

2 cups water

Heat oil (high-medium) in deep sauté pan. Sauté garlic for 10 minutes or until brown. Add garlic and green pepper, and continue cooking for another 5 minutes. Add all other ingredients and continue cooking for 10 minutes. Serves 2 to 4 people.

Blackened Tuna

2 tuna filets or steaks

3 tablespoons cold pressed olive oil

2 cloves garlic, chopped

1 teaspoon or more black pepper

1 teaspoon parsley

3 oz. baby spinach

Place the olive oil in a large sauté' pan at medium-high heat. Add the garlic and cook until slightly brown. Push the garlic to the edge around the pan. Add black pepper to both sides of the tuna. Place the tuna in the center of the pan. Add the other spices to everything in the pan. Cook the tuna until it is browned. Turn over and brown the other side. The tuna is done when the center is cooked. Serve over a bed of spinach. Serves two.

Chicken Cacciatore

3 tablespoons cold pressed olive oil

2 cloves garlic, chopped

1 onion, chopped (optional)

32 oz. tomato puree

1 whole chicken cut up in pieces

1 tablespoon oregano

1 tablespoon parsley

1/2 tablespoon sea salt

1/4 teaspoon black pepper

2 basil leaves

1 pound any vegetables you like except potatoes or carrots

Brown garlic in oil in a small fry pan. Put all ingredients together in an 8-quart pot. Simmer 1 hour, stirring every 15 minutes. Serves 4 people.

Chicken Casserole with Crushed Tomatoes

3 pounds thin sliced chicken breast (about 6 pieces)

2 cloves garlic, finely chopped

28 oz organic crushed plum tomatoes

3 tablespoons cold pressed olive oil

1/4 teaspoon sea salt

1/8 teaspoon fine black pepper

1 teaspoon parsley

6 fresh basil leaves, chopped

1 teaspoon oregano

Dash of cayenne pepper (optional)

Preheat oven to 350 F

Mix the above ingredients, except the chicken, in a bowl. Place a small amount of olive oil on the bottom of a covered Pyrex baking dish. Place the chicken breasts on the bottom of the dish. Pour over some tomato mixture. Add another layer of chicken breasts. Pour over more tomato mixture. Pour the remaining tomato mixture on the top layer. Cover and bake 90 minutes at 350 degrees F. Serves 6 people.

Chili

3 tablespoons cold pressed olive oil

2 cloves garlic, finely chopped

1 onion, chopped (optional)

1 green pepper, chopped

16 oz. tomatoes, finely chopped

16 oz. tomato puree

16 oz. white beans, drained

1 cup water

1 teaspoon basil

1/2 teaspoon black pepper

6 teaspoons chili powder

1 teaspoon oregano

1 teaspoon parsley

1/2 teaspoon sea salt

Heat oil in an 8-quart pot at medium heat. Sauté garlic, and peppers until brown. Add remaining ingredients. Cover and simmer for 60 minutes. Add more water if sauce is too thick. Serves 6 people.

Chopped Meat (Turkey) Allocca Style

2 tablespoons cold pressed olive oil

2 cloves garlic, chopped

1 onion, chopped (optional)

1/2 green pepper, finely chopped

16 oz. tomato puree

1 pound chopped turkey

1 teaspoon oregano

1/2 teaspoon parsley

1/2 teaspoon basil

1/2 teaspoon garlic powder

1/2 teaspoon sea salt

1/8 teaspoon black pepper

Dash cayenne pepper

Sauté garlic. Place remaining ingredients in a 4-quart pot, cover and cook for 10 -15 minutes over a medium heat, stirring frequently. Serve hot. Serves 2 people.

Curry Casserole

3 tablespoons cold pressed olive oil

2 cloves garlic, chopped

1 onion, chopped (optional)

16 oz. tomato puree

16 oz. lentils

1 head broccoli, chopped

1/2 teaspoon sea salt

1/2 teaspoon black pepper

1/2 teaspoon cardamom

A dash of cayenne, to your taste

1 teaspoon turmeric

1/2 teaspoon coriander

1/2 teaspoon cumin

In a 6-quart pot, sauté garlic in oil until slightly brown. Add rice and sauté for another minute. Add remaining ingredients. Bring to a boil. Cover, lower heat, and simmer for 45 minutes.

Healthy Salad

Romaine lettuce

Spinach

Cabbage, sliced

Red or green pepper, cut up

Bean sprouts

Mushrooms, sliced

Any additional vegetables you like except potatoes or carrots

Kale Casserole

2 tablespoons cold pressed olive oil

2 cloves garlic, chopped

1 onion, chopped (optional)

1 large bunch of kale, chopped

1 tablespoon lemon juice (not for migraineur's)

1/2 teaspoon sea salt

1/4 teaspoon black pepper

1 teaspoon basil

1/2 teaspoon parsley

1/2 teaspoon oregano

In a 6-quart pot, sauté garlic in oil until slightly brown. Add rice and sauté for another minute. Add remaining ingredients. Bring to a boil. Cover, lower heat, and simmer for 45 minutes.

Kale with Garlic and Oil

1 pound spinach pasta, cooked and drained

2 tablespoons cold pressed olive oil or more

2 cloves garlic, chopped

1 onion, chopped (optional)

1 bunch of kale, cut up

1/2 pound Shitaki mushrooms, sliced

1 teaspoon parsley

1 teaspoon oregano

1 teaspoon basil

1/2 teaspoon sea salt

1/8 teaspoon black pepper

Heat oil in a skillet. Add garlic, and mushrooms. Sauté until mushrooms and garlic are brown. Add remaining ingredients and sauté another 10 minutes. Serve over pasta. Serves 2 to 4 people.

Meat (Turkey) Loaf

2 tablespoons cold pressed olive oil

2 cloves garlic, chopped

1 onion, chopped (optional)

1 green pepper, chopped

1/2 pound fresh mushrooms, sliced

8 oz. tomato puree

2 pounds lean chopped turkey

1 tablespoon oregano

1/2 teaspoon parsley

1/2 teaspoon black pepper

1/2 teaspoon basil

1/2 teaspoon sea salt

2 teaspoons xantham gum

1/2 teaspoon agar agar

Sauté garlic till brown and put aside. Sauté mushrooms till brown and put aside. Mix all above ingredients except tomato sauce. Make into a load and cover with tomato sauce. Bake in oven at 425 degrees for 60 minutes. Serves 2 to 4 people

Portobella Casserole

2 tablespoons cold pressed olive oil or more

2 cloves garlic, chopped

1 onion, chopped (optional)

1 pound Portabella mushrooms, diced into 3/4" squares

3-1/2 cups water

6 oz. baby spinach

1/2 teaspoon sea salt

1/4 teaspoon black pepper

1 teaspoon basil

1/2 teaspoon parsley

1/2 teaspoon oregano

In a 6-quart pot, sauté garlic in oil until slightly brown. Add mushrooms and sauté for another 5 minutes. Add rice and sauté for another minute. Add remaining ingredients. Bring to a boil. Cover, lower heat, and simmer for 45 minutes.

Roasted Chicken

Preheat the oven to 350 degrees F.

Oil the bottom of a large poultry pan with v-shaped rack. Place cut potatoes and carrots on the bottom of the pan. Place cut onions and carrots on top of the potatoes. Sprinkle with cold pressed olive oil, sea salt (small amount), black pepper, parsley, basil, and oregano. Place the chicken on the v-shaped rack. Approximate cooking times (20 minutes per pound plus an additional 20 minutes):

3 pounds = 1 hour, 20 minutes
3.5 pounds = 1 hour, 30 minutes
4 pounds = 1 hour, 40 minutes
5 pounds = 2 hours
6 pounds = 2 hours, 20 minutes
7 pounds = 2 hours, 40 minutes
8 pounds = 3 hours minutes

Note: if two chickens are used, calculate the time for the weight of the larger chicken and add 30 minutes.

Note: if the chicken(s) were frozen and not fully thawed, add 30 minutes to the cooking time.

The roasting pan recommended is the "Rachael Ray Oven Lovin' Non-Stick 10" x 14" Roaster with V-Rack." The non-stock pan and rack make it is easy to clean. Two 3.5 pound chickens can fit in this pan.

Sausage (Chicken) with Onions and Peppers

2 pounds chicken sausage
2 tablespoons cold pressed olive oil
2 onions, chopped
2 bell peppers, chopped
1 teaspoon parsley
1 teaspoon oregano
1 teaspoon basil
1/2 teaspoon sea salt
1/8 teaspoon black pepper

In a 6-quart pot, add the oil, onions, and peppers. Cook covered over medium heat for 5 minutes. Add the sausages and continue cooking covered for 20 minutes or until done. Serves 2 to 4 people.

Salmon or Tuna – Allocca Style

2 tablespoons cold pressed olive oil or more

2 cloves garlic, chopped

2 salmon or tuna filets

1/2 teaspoon black pepper

1/4 teaspoon sea salt

1 teaspoon parsley

6 fresh basil leaves, chopped

3 oz. fresh organic baby spinach

Remove the skin from the filet using a paper towel to grip it. Place the olive oil in a large sauté pan at medium-high heat. Add the garlic and cook until slightly brown. Push the garlic to the edge around the pan. Place the salmon filet in the center of the pan. Add basil to the garlic around the edge of the pan. Add the other spices to everything in the pan. Cook the salmon until it is browned. Turn over and brown the other side. The salmon is done when the center is white. Serve over a bed of spinach. Serves two.

Stuffed Chicken with Mushrooms

1 pound portabella or button mushrooms, chopped

2 tablespoons cold pressed olive oil

1/2 teaspoon sea salt

1/4 teaspoon black pepper

Dash of cayenne pepper

1/2 teaspoon parsley

1/2 teaspoon basil

1/2 teaspoon oregano

2 cloves garlic, chopped

1 onion, chopped (optional)

3 pounds (10 slices) thin-sliced chicken breast

Sauté mushrooms in oil for 5 minutes. Add herbs and spices and set aside. Place 5 thin-sliced chicken breasts into an oiled 15 x 10 x 2 Pyrex dish. Add some mushroom mixture to each slice. Next, place another 5 thin-sliced chicken breast on top of each of the previously filled breasts. Add the remaining mixture on top of each thin-sliced chicken breast. Place in the oven and low broil for 35 minutes.

Stuffed Chicken with Tomatoes and Olives

16 oz tomato puree

16 oz black olives, chopped

2 tablespoons cold pressed olive oil

1/2 teaspoon sea salt

1/4 teaspoon black pepper

Dash of cayenne pepper

1/2 teaspoon parsley

1/2 teaspoon basil

1/2 teaspoon oregano

1/2 teaspoon garlic powder

3 pounds (10 slices) thin-sliced chicken breast

Mix the tomatoes, olives, herbs, and spices in a bowl and set aside. Place 5 thin-sliced chicken breasts into an oiled 15 x 10 x 2 Pyrex dish. Add some tomato and olive mixture to each slice. Next, place another 5 thin-sliced chicken breast on top of each of the previously filled breasts. Add the remaining mixture on top of each thin-sliced chicken breast. Place in the oven and low broil for 35 minutes.

Turkey

Preheat the oven to 400 degrees F.

Place cut potatoes and place them on the bottom of a large poultry pan with v-shaped rack. Place cut carrots onions on top of the potatoes. Sprinkle with cold pressed olive oil, sea salt (small amount), black pepper, and garlic powder.

Place the turkey on the v-shaped rack.

Make a batter of olive oil, melted butter (small amount), sea salt (small amount), and black pepper. Inject the batter into the turkey.

Make a "tent" out of aluminum foil and place it loosely over the turkey to keep it moist.

Cook the turkey for 1 hour. Lower the temperature to 350 degrees F.

Insert a cooking thermometer into the breast of the turkey. Cook the turkey until it reaches 165 degrees F. Approximate cooking times:

10 pounds = 3 to 3-1/2 hours

15 pounds = 3-1/2 to 4 hours

20 pounds = 4 to 4-1/2 hours (feeds 10 people)

25 pounds = 4-1/2 to 5 hours

30 pounds = 5 to 5-1/2 hours

Remove the aluminum foil tent 1 hour before the turkey is cooked to brown the skin.

Vegetable Casserole

2 tablespoons cold pressed olive oil

2 cloves garlic, chopped

1 onion, chopped (optional)

1 red pepper, chopped

1/2 pound mushrooms, sliced

1 cup lentils, cooked

16 oz. tomatoes, finely chopped

Vegetables, chopped (spinach, bok choy, kale, etc.)

1 teaspoon basil

1/2 teaspoon black pepper

Dash of cayenne pepper

1 teaspoon garlic powder

1 teaspoon oregano

1 teaspoon parsley

1 teaspoon sea salt

In a 8-quart pot, sauté garlic, peppers, and mushrooms. Add remaining ingredients. Bring to a boil. Cover and simmer for 45 minutes. Serves 6 to 8 people.

Baked French Fries

Preheat oven 400 degrees F.

4-5 medium sized potatoes, 2 pounds, washed and dried (do not peel).

Okay, they are not fried. But, they taste great and they are healthy too! Wrap the potatoes in wax paper. Cook in a microwave oven for 1.5 minutes on high. Unwrap and insert each potato into the potato slicer creating french fry cuts. Sprinkle rosemary leaves on top. Place the cuts onto a french fry baking sheet (with holes) and bake in a conventional oven for 45 minutes at 400 degrees F or until golden brown or darker if you prefer.

From www.chefscatalog.com

Progressive Deluxe French Fry Cutter, Item # 26027, $34.95

CHEFS Nonstick French Fry Baking Sheet, Item # 29319, $24.95

Broccoli with Tomato Sauce

2 tablespoons cold pressed olive oil

2 cloves garlic, chopped

1 onion, chopped (optional)

1 large head of broccoli tips

32 oz. tomato puree

1 teaspoon oregano

1 teaspoon parsley

1/2 teaspoon sea salt

1/8 teaspoon black pepper

1 basil leaf

Sauté garlic in oil. Add garlic and brown. Put all ingredients together in a 6-quart pot. Simmer 30 minutes Serve over rice.

Dahl

1 tablespoon cold pressed olive oil

2 cloves garlic, chopped

1/2 cup water or more

1/2 teaspoon black pepper

1/2 teaspoon cardamom

A dash or more of cayenne

1 teaspoon turmeric

1/2 teaspoon coriander

1/2 teaspoon cumin

1/2 teaspoon sea salt

16 oz. lentils

Sauté garlic and oil in a 3-quart pot. Add remaining ingredients. Bring to a boil. Simmer for 30 minutes.

Lentil Salad

Lentils are high in protein and fiber. Fiber will promote bowel movements.

2 cups dry green or brown lentils

4 cups water

1 tablespoon cold pressed olive oil

1/4 teaspoon garlic powder

1/2 teaspoon parsley

1/2 teaspoon basil

1/2 teaspoon oregano

dash of sea salt

dash of black pepper

Place lentils and water in a 4-quart saucepan. Bring to a boil. Reduce heat, cover, and simmer for 40 minutes or until done. Allow the beans to cool. Then add the remaining ingredients.

Mushrooms in Garlic & Oil

2 tablespoons cold pressed olive oil

2 cloves garlic, chopped

1 onion, chopped (optional)

1 pound shitaki or portabello mushrooms, sliced

1 teaspoon parsley

1 teaspoon oregano

1 teaspoon basil

1/2 teaspoon sea salt

1/8 teaspoon black pepper

Heat oil in a skillet. Add garlic and mushrooms. Sauté until mushrooms and garlic are brown. Add remaining ingredients and sauté another 10 minutes.

Oil and Lemon Dressing

1/4 cup lemon juice (not for migraineur's)

1/2 cup cold pressed olive oil

1/2 teaspoon basil

1/2 teaspoon parsley

1 teaspoon oregano

1/2 teaspoon garlic powder

1/8 teaspoon black pepper

1/4 teaspoon sea salt

Mix all ingredients together in a jar or container. Shake well just before using.

Squash

2 pound butternut squash

2 tablespoons cold pressed olive oil

2 cloves of garlic, finely chopped

4 scallions, chopped

1 leek, sliced

1/2 teaspoon sea salt

1/4 teaspoon black pepper

1 pound rice pasta

Peel the butternut squash. Cut the squash into 4 sections length-wise. Remove the seeds. Slice each section into 1/4" slices. Set aside squash. Begin boiling the water for the pasta. At medium heat, add the garlic to a 6-quart pot and sauté until slightly brown. Add the scallions and cook for another minute. Add the leek and cook for another minute. Add the squash and lower heat. Cover and simmer for 20 to 30 minutes or until the squash is tender. Stir occasionally. Serve separately or over pasta or rice.

Steamed Vegetables

6 pieces of broccoli tips

3 slices of cabbage, cut up

2 pieces of kale, cut up

Any additional vegetables you like except potatoes or carrots

1/2 teaspoon basil

1/2 teaspoon parsley

1/2 teaspoon oregano

1/2 teaspoon sea salt

1 tablespoon cold pressed olive oil

Place potatoes and cabbage in steamer pot and steam for 15 minutes. Add the rest of the ingredients and steam for an additional 5 minutes. For microwave: cover all vegetables and cook for 10 minutes) Add spices as desired.

Stuffed Artichokes

1 tablespoon cold pressed olive oil

2 cloves garlic, finely chopped

6 large-size artichokes

1 teaspoon basil

1 teaspoon parsley

1 teaspoon oregano

1/4 teaspoon sea salt

1/8 teaspoon black pepper

Cut off artichoke stems and trim 1/2 inch from tops of leaves. Separate leaves slightly to allow for stuffing. Sauté garlic and oil until brown. In a large bowl mix together above ingredients. Spoon mixture into the artichokes and place in a steamer pot and steam for 30 minutes at medium heat.

Tossed Salad

Arugula and/or baby spinach

Endive

Radicchio

Garbanzo beans

Oil and lemon dressing

Use quantities of the above appropriate for the number of people being served.

Bread and Muffins

Banana Nut Muffins

Preheat oven to 350 F

2 cups brown rice flour

1 cup tapioca flour

2 tablespoons potato starch flour

2 tablespoons baking powder (non-aluminum)

2 tablespoons fructose or 1/8 teaspoon Stevia powder

2 teaspoons xantham gum

1/2 teaspoon agar agar

1/2 teaspoon sea salt

4 medium fresh almost green bananas, peeled & mashed

3/4 cup almonds or walnuts, chopped

1-3/4 cups rice milk or water or organic cow's milk

2 tablespoons cold pressed sunflower oil

1 teaspoon vanilla flavor (non-alcoholic)

Mix dry ingredients with electric mixer. Slowly add the milk while mixing. Add canola oil and vanilla. Add bananas. Spoon mixture into an oiled muffin pan. Bake at 350 F for 45 minutes or until top is light brown. Remove muffins from the pan and cool on a cake rack. Makes 12 muffins.

Blueberry Muffins

Preheat oven to 350 F

2 cups brown rice flour

1 cup tapioca flour

2 tablespoons potato starch flour

2 tablespoons baking powder (non-aluminum)

3 tablespoons fructose or 3/16 teaspoon Stevia powder

2 teaspoons xantham gum

1/2 teaspoon agar agar

1/2 teaspoon sea salt

1-3/4 cups rice milk or water or organic cow's milk

2 tablespoons cold pressed sunflower oil

1 teaspoon vanilla flavor (non-alcoholic)

1 cup blueberries or other fruit

Mix dry ingredients with electric mixer. Slowly add the milk while mixing. Add canola oil and vanilla. Add blueberries. Spoon mixture into an oiled muffin pan. Bake at 350 F for 40 minutes or until top is light brown. Remove muffins from the pan and cool on a cake rack. Makes 9 muffins. Add a little water to the unused muffin spaces.

Brown Rice Bread

Preheat oven to 350 F

2 cups brown rice flour

1 cup tapioca flour

2 tablespoons potato starch flour

2 tablespoons baking powder (non-aluminum)

2 tablespoons fructose or 1/8 teaspoon Stevia powder

2 teaspoons xantham gum

1 teaspoon agar agar

1/2 teaspoon sea salt

1-1/4 cups rice milk or water or organic cow's milk

1 tablespoon cold pressed olive oil

Mix dry ingredients with dough hooks. Slowly add the milk while kneading. Add olive oil. Dough will be slightly sticky. Press into an oiled loaf pan with a lightly oiled spatula. Bake at 350 F for 60 minutes or until top is medium brown. Remove from the pan and cool on a cake rack. Variations, add 2 teaspoons of Italian seasoning or other seasoning to your taste.

Brown Rice Foccacia Bread

Preheat oven to 400 F

1 cup brown rice flour

1/2 cup tapioca flour

1 tablespoon potato starch flour

1 tablespoon baking powder (non-aluminum)

1 tablespoon fructose or 1/16 teaspoon Stevia powder

2 teaspoons xantham gum

1/2 teaspoon agar agar

1/4 teaspoon sea salt

3/4 cup rice milk or water or organic cow's milk

1/2 tablespoon cold pressed olive oil

2 cloves garlic, pressed

Mix dry ingredients with dough hooks. Slowly add the milk while kneading. Add olive oil. Dough will be slightly sticky. Press into an oiled 8-inch baking pan with a lightly oiled spatula. Brush top with olive oil. Add garlic, salt, pepper, oregano, fresh basil, thinly sliced tomato. Bake at 400 F for 25 minutes or until crust is medium brown. Remove from the pan and cool on a cake rack.

Corn Muffins

Preheat oven to 350 F

2 cups yellow corn meal

1/2 cup brown rice flour

1/2 cup tapioca flour

2 tablespoons potato starch flour

2 tablespoons baking powder (non-aluminum)

3 tablespoons fructose or 3/16 teaspoon Stevia powder

2 teaspoons xantham gum

1/2 teaspoon agar agar

1/2 teaspoon sea salt

1-3/4 cups rice or coconut milk

2 tablespoons cold pressed sunflower oil

1 teaspoon vanilla flavor (non-alcoholic)

1 cup corn kernels (optional)

Mix dry ingredients with electric mixer. Slowly add the milk while mixing. Add canola oil and vanilla. Add optional corn kernels. Spoon mixture into an oiled muffin pan. Bake at 350 F for 40 minutes or until top is light brown. Remove muffins from the pan and cool on a cake rack. Makes 9 muffins. Add a little water to the unused muffin spaces.

Almond Cookies and Pancakes

Preheat oven to 350 F. 3 cups almond flour

1 cup cashew nuts - coarsely chopped

1/2 cup sesame seeds

2 teaspoons baking powder (non-aluminum) (2 tablespoons for pancakes)

2 teaspoons ground cinnamon

1 teaspoon ground nutmeg

1/2 teaspoon sea salt

1/2 cup cold pressed sunflower oil

2 teaspoons xantham gum

1/2 teaspoon agar agar

1/4 cup water (1/2 cup for pancakes)

Organic butter to spread

Mix dry ingredients, then add liquids & mix well. Spoon out onto a lightly oiled cookie sheet with a tablespoon or medium size ice cream scoop. Then, flatten slightly. Bake 30 minutes or until slightly brown. Cool on a wire rack. Makes approximately 26 cookies. Turn the cookie upside down and add butter. 7.6 Carbohydrates per cookie (35 g).

Apple Cashew Dessert

3 medium peeled and sliced apples (390 grams, 50.9 grams carbohydrate)

1-1/4 cups filtered water

1 cup cashew nuts (139 grams, 39.7 grams carbohydrate)

1 cup cashew flour (107 grams, 30.6 grams carbohydrate)

4 tablespoons unsweetened shredded coconut (2.3 grams carbohydrate)

4 fresh organic strawberries, sliced

Cinnamon

Place all ingredients into a 4-quart saucepan and cook at medium heat for 10 minutes or until the apples are soft. Place the mixture into four 8 oz pyrex cups. Place one sliced strawberry on top of each cup. Sprinkle cinnamon on top of each cup. Refrigerate and serve cold.

Carbohydrate contents = 130.4 grams divided by 4 = 32.6 grams per serving.

Brown Rice Pudding

1 cup brown rice

1/4 cup fructose

1/4 teaspoon sea salt

2 teaspoons agar agar

1 teaspoon cinnamon

1 teaspoon almond flavor (non-alcoholic)

6 cups rice or coconut milk o rwater

     Place ingredients into a 4-quart pot and bring to a boil. Cover and simmer for 2 hours. Pour into Pyrex cups and refrigerate.

Carrot Cake

Preheat oven to 350 F.

2 cups brown rice flour

1 cup tapioca flour

2 tablespoons potato starch flour

2 teaspoons xantham gum

1 teaspoon agar agar

2 tablespoons baking powder (non-aluminum)

2 teaspoons cinnamon

1 teaspoon salt

1 cup fructose

1/2 cup almonds, chopped

1 cup shredded coconut

2 cups carrots, grated

1 cup cold pressed sunflower oil

1 3/4 cups or more of rice or coconut milk

3 teaspoons almond extract

     Combine dry ingredients together. Add liquid ingredients and mix. Add a little water if the mixture is too dry. Put into a 9 x 9 inch oiled pan and bake at 350 F for 45 minutes.

Carob Brownies

Preheat oven 350 degrees F.

2 cups brown rice flour

1 cup tapioca flour

2 tablespoons potato starch flour

2 tablespoons baking powder (non-aluminum)

2 teaspoons xantham gum

1 teaspoon agar agar

1-1/4 cups carob powder

1 cup shredded coconut

1 cup carob chips

1/2 teaspoon sea salt

1 cup walnuts or almonds, coarsely, chopped

2 tablespoons cold pressed sunflower oil

1/2 cup fructose

2 teaspoons vanilla flavor (non-alcoholic)

1 3/4 cups or more of rice or coconut milk or water

Mix dry ingredients. Add liquid ingredients and mix well for a slightly loose mixture. Pour into an oiled 10 x 15 Pyrex baking pan and spread evenly. Bake 40 minutes. Allow to cool completely. Cut into squares and remove from baking dish.

Cashew Cookies and Pancakes

Preheat oven to 350 F. 3 cups cashew flour

1 cup cashew nuts - coarsely chopped

1/2 cup sesame seeds

2 teaspoons baking powder (non-aluminum) (2 tablespoons for pancakes)

2 teaspoons ground cinnamon

1 teaspoon ground nutmeg

1/2 teaspoon sea salt

1/2 cup cold pressed sunflower oil

2 teaspoons xantham gum

1 teaspoon agar agar

1/4 cup water (1/2 cup for pancakes)

Organic butter to spread

Mix dry ingredients, then add liquids & mix well. Spoon out onto a lightly oiled cookie sheet with a tablespoon or medium size ice cream scoop. Then, flatten slightly. Bake 30 minutes or until slightly brown. Cool on a wire rack. Makes approximately 26 cookies. Turn the cookie upside down and add butter. 8.5 Carbohydrates per cookie (35 g).

Coconut Icing

1/2 cup cold pressed sunflower oil

1/2 cup rice or coconut milk

2 tablespoons fructose

1-2 cups shredded coconut (to make thick)

     In a blender, mix all ingredients on high for 3 minutes. Apply to the cake with a spatula.

Pie Crust

Preheat oven to 350 F

1 cup yellow corn meal

1/4 cup brown rice flour

1/4 cup tapioca flour

1 tablespoon potato starch flour

1 teaspoon baking powder (non-aluminum)

2 tablespoons fructose

2 teaspoons xantham gum

1 teaspoon agar agar

1/4 teaspoon sea salt

1/2 cup rice or coconut milk or water

3 tablespoons cold pressed sunflower oil

1/2 teaspoon vanilla flavor (non-alcoholic)

     Mix dry ingredients with electric mixer. Slowly add rice milk while mixing. Add canola oil and vanilla. Press into an oiled baking pie plate with a lightly oiled spatula. Add filling and bake at 350 F for 50 minutes or until crust is light brown. Allow to cool completely before serving.

Pie Filling - Apple

2 large apples, peeled and sliced

3/4 cup water

1 teaspoon lemon juice

1 teaspoon cinnamon

1/2 teaspoon nutmeg

2 teaspoons agar agar

     Cover and simmer on low heat for 2 minutes. Add to pie crust.

Pie Filling - Blueberry

16 oz blueberries

3/4 cup water

2 teaspoons agar agar

     Cover and simmer on low heat for 2 minutes. Add to pie crust.

Pumpkin Pudding or Pie Filling

2 cups pumpkin or squash, cooked

1/4 cup fructose or 1/2 teaspoon Stevia powder

1 teaspoon vanilla flavor (non-alcoholic)

1 teaspoon cinnamon

1/2 teaspoon nutmeg

1/2 teaspoon ground ginger

1/4 teaspoon ground cloves

2 teaspoons agar agar

1 cup rice or coconut milk or water

     Simmer ingredients in a 4-quart pot. Stir until mixture is well blended. Pour into pyrex cups, then refrigerate. If used as a pie filling, you do not need to simmer the mixture – add to pie crust.

Biometabolic Analysis

Have Your Patients Feel Great and Live Longer through Biometabolic Analysis

It all started with a solution to migraine headaches. Then, more solutions were created. A biochemical model reveals the complex mechanisms of a biological process. The first biochemical model Dr. Allocca created revealed the mechanisms of migraine headaches. Research progressed to developing biochemical models for depression, insomnia, bipolar disorder, violence, carbohydrate craving, membrane transport systems, and much more. Then, Dr. Allocca programmed these complex biochemical models into a state-of-the-art software program, which is called "Biometabolic Analysis." The software program has evolved and is constantly evolving since 1996.

One of the most important biochemical models in biometabolic Analysis is the transport of nutrients from the blood stream into the cells, which may not happen automatically. People may be eating right and getting plenty of exercise, but if the critical process of transporting nutrients into the cells is not taking place, problems can occur. For example, lactic acid can build up inside the cells damaging the cell membranes and DNA. This is why the body ages, organs degrade, and diseases begin. Biometabolic analysis can determine if this is occurring and facilitate the appropriate changes. Most of the biochemical models used in the program are published in Dr. Allocca's textbooks.

Biometabolic Analysis produces an individualized step-by-step plan geared towards each person's needs to facilitate the appropriate changes for problems discovered.

Most cases often have additional complications. Biometabolic Analysis address those complications.

Parameters Analyzed

Age

Sex

Height and Weight

Blood Pressure

Urinalysis

Zinc Taste Test

Daytime Core Temperature

Saliva pH

Bioelectric Impedance Analysis

Vascular Sonography: brachial and posterior tibial

Pulse Oximetry

Symptoms Questionnaire

Biometabolic Analysis Report

Client Information

Conditions which may Interfere with Good Health

Basal Metabolic Rate

Body Mass Index

Test Results Analyzed and Explained

Symptoms Probability Profile

Supplemental Information

Food and Supplement Recommendations

Problems Addressed

Migraine Prevention

Depression

Insomnia

Bipolar disorder

Excessive Aggression

Anger and Violence

Decreased Sexuality

Carbohydrate Craving

Increased Body Temperature

Irritable Bowel Syndrome

Tinnitus

Fibromyalgia

Premenstrual Syndrome

Seasonal Affective Disorder

Weight Problems

Poor Digestion and Malabsorption

Hormonal Imbalances

Irritable Bowel Syndrome

Intestinal Candida (yeast) Overgrowth

Allergies

Pre and Post Menopausal Syndrome

Nutritional Deficiencies

Inflammation

Arthritis

Adrenal Imbalances

Thyroid Imbalances

Diabetes

Peripheral Arterial Disease

and much more...

For more information, see www.allocca.com.